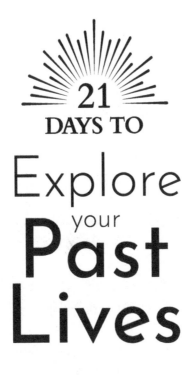

21
DAYS TO
Explore
your
Past
Lives

Also in the 21 Days series

21 Days to Awaken the Writer Within
by Lisa Fugard

21 Days to Become a Money Magnet
by Marie-Claire Carlyle

21 Days to Decode Your Dreams
by Leon Nacson

21 Days to Find Success and Inner Peace
by Dr. Wayne W. Dyer

21 Days to Master Numerology
by David A. Phillips

21 Days to Understand Qabalah
by David Wells

21 Days to Unlock the Power of Affirmations
by Louise Hay

21 Days to Work with Crystals
by Judy Hall

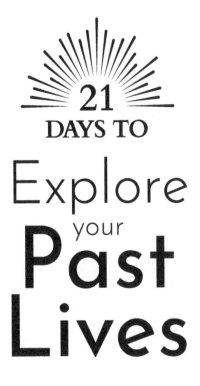

21
DAYS TO

Explore
your
Past
Lives

Release Ancient Trauma, Find True Healing,
and Listen to the Secrets of Your Soul

DENISE LINN

HAY HOUSE

Carlsbad, California • New York City
London • Sydney • New Delhi

Published in the United Kingdom by:
Hay House UK Ltd, The Sixth Floor, Watson House,
54 Baker Street, London W1U 7BU
Tel: +44 (0)20 3927 7290; www.hayhouse.co.uk

Published in the United States of America by:
Hay House Inc., PO Box 5100, Carlsbad, CA 92018-5100
Tel: (1) 760 431 7695 or (800) 654 5126; www.hayhouse.com

Published in Australia by:
Hay House Australia Pty Ltd, 18/36 Ralph St, Alexandria NSW 2015
Tel: (61) 2 9669 4299; www.hayhouse.com.au

Published in India by:
Hay House Publishers India, Muskaan Complex,
Plot No.3, B-2, Vasant Kunj, New Delhi 110 070
Tel: (91) 11 4176 1620; www.hayhouse.co.in

Text © Denise Linn, 2011, 2023

21 Days to Explore Your Past Lives draws from Denise Linn's best-selling *Past Lives, Present Miracles* (Hay House, 2008).

The moral rights of the author have been asserted.

The information given in this book should not be treated as a substitute for professional medical advice; always consult a medical practitioner. Any use of information in this book is at the reader's discretion and risk. Neither the author nor the publisher can be held responsible for any loss, claim or damage arising out of the use, or misuse, of the suggestions made, the failure to take medical advice or for any material on third-party websites.

A catalogue record for this book is available from the British Library.

Tradepaper ISBN: 978-1-78817-905-8
E-book ISBN: 978-1-78817-923-2
Audiobook ISBN: 978-1-78817-864-8

Printed in Great Britain by Clays Ltd, Elcograf S.p.A.

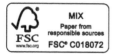

Contents

Publisher's Note   vii

Introduction   ix

Day 1: Why Past-life Therapy Works   1

Day 2: Reincarnation   9

Day 3: Soul Mates and Love Mates   15

Day 4: Karma, Destiny, and Free Will   23

Day 5: Are Past Lives Real?   33

Day 6: How to Discover Who You Were   39

Day 7: Clues from Your Childhood   45

Day 8: Clues from Your Tastes   53

Day 9: Clues from Your Name and Your   63
            Characteristics

Day 10: Clues from Your Body and Your Health   73

Day 11: Clues from Your Relationships   81

Day 12: Clues from Places, Events, Cultures,   89
and Déjà Vu

Day 13: Dreams and Past Lives   97

Day 14: Remembering and Analyzing   105
Your Dreams

Day 15: Using the Power of Creative   113
Visualization

Day 16: The Inner Voyage: A Past-life   121
Visualization Technique

Day 17: The Inner Voyage Meditation   131

Day 18: How to Heal Past-life Blockages   137
with Regression: Method 1

Day 19: How to Heal Past-life Blockages   145
with Regression: Methods 2 and 3

Day 20: How to Heal Past-life Blockages   153
with Regression: Method 4

Day 21: Looking Forward: Time and   161
Future Lives

Afterword   171
About the Author   175

Publisher's Note

Research has shown that establishing a habit requires 21 days' practice. That's why Hay House has decided to adapt the work of some of its most prestigious authors into these short, 21-day courses, designed specifically to develop new mastery of subjects such as past lives.

21 Days to Explore Your Past Lives draws from Denise Linn's best-selling *Past Lives, Present Miracles* (Hay House, 2008).

Other titles that will help you to further explore the concepts featured in the 21-day program are listed at the beginning of this book.

Introduction

You can create extraordinary positive change in your life, smoothly and effortlessly. It's simply a matter of remembering who you are—and in order to do this, you must clear the blockages that stand between you and your soul. Almost all of these obstacles have their roots in your far past, so it's immensely valuable to travel back into time to release them. However, most of us are so caught up in limiting beliefs about who we are and what we deserve that it's almost impossible to take that journey.

If you really want to know who you are, and you're ready for your life to blossom, this book will reveal secret pathways that will help you clear your inner clutter so that you can truly discover why you're here. With this knowledge, you'll learn how to manifest your innermost dreams. The time is now! You wouldn't be reading this book if you weren't prepared to begin the journey.

As the transformation of our planet intensifies, exploring past lives can be an increasing source of healing and inspiration. But how can you best take advantage of the energies now available for growth and personal expansion? In what ways can you remember who you were in your former lives and then release any negative programming that has carried forward into your present life? How does releasing blockages from the past help you create miracles in your current existence? What should you do so that you can remember your dreams and understand what they're trying to tell you? Why is this a very significant time in history? In the following chapters, I'll give you the simple, viable answers and solutions.

This book offers easy-to-use techniques to help you recall events from your previous lives. It also explains reincarnation and karma, and why these concepts are so important at this time. You'll learn how to use a range of past-life clues to discover who you were in earlier incarnations. As our planet's vibratory rate continues to accelerate, it's vital that you listen to the secrets of your soul. I'll teach you how to program, remember, and interpret these messages.

Right now in our human evolution, massive, exciting changes that have been foretold by native cultures around the world are beginning to occur on many levels. The aim of this book is to provide you with information and techniques that will show you how to release the past so that you can experience joy in your everyday life and prepare for upcoming events.

We are the spiritual heirs of the planet. If we can let go of the ancient blockages and limitations from the past and listen to the inner guidance of our soul, we can lovingly step into the future.

DAY 1

Why Past-life Therapy Works

Today we are going to look at why exploring our past lives can help us in our present lives.

Past-life therapy is healing because it allows you to get to the source of your problems; until then, you're dealing with symptoms rather than causes. Whether you call it genetic coding, cellular memory, or even collective unconsciousness, the vast repository of our previous experiences rules us all; and in many ways, these experiences dictate the situations we encounter in the present.

For example, many compulsions and phobias are rooted in the distant past. If you've always hated wearing anything tight around your neck, you may discover that you were choked to death in a previous lifetime. By reliving—and healing—ancient memories and associated emotions, your current life-limiting behaviors will change.

We often create incidents today that subconsciously remind us of events from our former lives, in an attempt to heal the original pain. If emotions such as fear, anger, or grief were suppressed during traumatic events in a past life, they'll stay embedded in your energy field and form inner conflicts that recur lifetime after lifetime. As you continue to push these undesired feelings deeper into your psyche, a greater barrier builds between you and whatever you're afraid to confront. But when you relive a past-life incident, the emotions and decisions that were held back for so long finally have the opportunity to rise to the surface and be released so that they no longer control you.

To understand why past-life therapy works, it's important to realize that it's not necessarily what you endured in your earlier lives that creates problems in your present life; rather, it's the trauma and emotions that you suppressed in the past that initiates difficulties in the present. Your past experiences don't cause continuing problems—it's your reactions to them that create challenges. For example, suffering a fatal wound in a former life won't necessarily create a blockage in your present life, but a fatal wound while feeling suppressed intense emotional anguish could.

Imagine two similar scenarios. In the first, an Aztec warrior is fighting alongside his best friend. The dust is churning as spears fly on either side of the gallant warrior. Suddenly in the haze of battle, a spear is flung straight at the chest of his friend. The young warrior steps in front of it, valiantly saving the life of his comrade. Mortally wounded by the spear that pierced his chest, he dies but feels a deep peace, for he has saved his friend's life.

In the second scenario, two young warriors are battling side by side. They are best friends. Suddenly in the thrall of battle and obscured by thick haze and dust, one turns to the other and thrusts a spear into his friend's chest. As the warrior lies dying on the battlefield, he learns that his best friend is having an affair with his wife and wants him out of the way. He dies making a decision that he can never really trust anyone.

In both scenes the physical trauma is the same—a spear wound to the chest causes death. In the first instance, the Aztec warrior feels exhilaration at having spared the life of his friend. In the second scenario, however, the warrior decides that it's unwise to trust anyone. In future lives, whenever this man begins to get close to someone, similar memories and decisions will be activated. Whenever he starts to trust, he experiences severe chest pains and the fear of being betrayed. For him, establishing a bond with another activates an emotional and physical response from a past life.

So it's not your past-life trauma that causes your present-day blockages; it's the meaning you give to those events that haunts you through time. And it's possible to travel back and change the significance of any event, and thus create a time/space domino effect that transforms your present life.

One of the most powerful things that you can gain from past-life therapy is forgiveness. In order to heal, you must be willing to forgive the past. It's much easier to pardon those who have hurt you in your present life once you understand the karma that precipitated the situation. When you travel to the past-life source of your hurt—to absolve yourself and others—a loving energy weaves its way through time and space to your current life. Of course it's important to forgive those who hurt or denied you in a previous lifetime; however, it's just as vital to release the guilt for things that you did to others. (If you have difficulty letting go, you must forgive yourself for not forgiving.)

Some of the most rewarding comments I receive after past-life seminars relate to forgiving present- and past-life circumstances. In Australia, I conducted a seminar at the Japanese-owned Nikko Hotel, and a woman who attended that seminar later wrote me an interesting letter. Upon entering the hotel, she experienced an intense wave of resentment and panic washing over her. She almost fled but was very glad that she stayed because a debilitating condition, which she'd had since she was a teenager, totally healed.

In her letter, she told me that when she was 17 years old, she had been taken prisoner in Indonesia by Japanese soldiers during World War II. She wrote: "I suffered physically as well as mentally from their brutality. I survived, but my intestines were damaged from untreated dysentery. I was severely undernourished, and I harbored a deep hatred for everything Japanese. I've sought treatment from many physicians and psychologists during the last 50 years, but I've had to live with a chronic weakness of the bowel and a constant pain in the solar plexus."

She had come to see her suffering as something that she carried for all reviled people in the world. The woman went on to tell me that after she'd regressed to a past life in my seminar, she was able to observe the source of her current resentment (she didn't mention what the past life was). As a result of forgiving prior-life circumstances, the pain that had plagued her for 50 years had completely lifted! "My debilitating pain disappeared during the seminar, and today I'm still free of it! When I left the hotel, I even gave a friendly greeting to the Japanese staff," she wrote. She added that she had spent time talking to some of them and found them to be very pleasant, lovely people: "I feel free! Free from pain! Free from all animosity and all resentment! Truly and gloriously free and easy!"

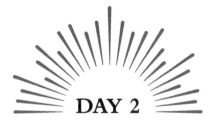

DAY 2

Reincarnation

Today we are going to explore the concept of reincarnation, which is the center of past-life therapy. Reincarnation has been with us since before recorded history. It's the doctrine or belief that an essential part—the higher self, or the soul—of each human being survives death and is reborn in another body. Although a new identity develops in each life, there's a spiritual part of the being that remains constant throughout successive lives.

Current estimates suggest that at least a third of the people alive today believe that the soul is eternal and repeatedly returns to Earth through rebirth into new bodies in order to grow and learn. A recent Harris Poll of the spiritual beliefs of Americans found that 27 percent believe in reincarnation—that is, they believe they were once another person. This includes 40 percent of people aged 25 to 29 but only 14 percent of individuals aged 65 and over (which indicates that the belief in reincarnation is growing among our youth).

The spiritual belief in an enduring "self" that incarnates again and again declares that each lifetime provides a wealth of experiences that allow us as divine beings to become stronger, more balanced, and more loving. And eventually, we reunite with Spirit. (At times I prefer to use the words Spirit or Creator instead of God because some people equate God with a male deity in the sky who's judgmental. To me, the words God, Goddess, the Creator, Great Spirit, Spirit, and Cosmic Consciousness all mean the same thing—which is the living force within all things.)

Spontaneous reincarnation episodes can occur in many ways. Have you ever had the eerie experience of being in a strange town and feeling a sense of recognition almost too deep to describe? Have you ever heard a particular piece of music and felt transported by it or had a vivid dream about a time in history or a foreign country that seemed extraordinarily familiar and real? All these incidents could have their roots in past lifetimes.

In one life, perhaps you were very poor and thus had a chance to learn humility and resourcefulness firsthand. In another, you might have been wealthy in order to understand how to deal with money fairly and positively. You may have been blind in order to activate your inner sight, or athletic to experience and comprehend physical strength. You might have been a woman in one life and a man in another—or Caucasian in one and Asian in another. Try to think of past lives not so much as building blocks but as pieces of a jigsaw puzzle, with each piece a lifetime making you more balanced.

Throughout history, great thinkers have pondered the mysteries of life, birth, and rebirth. The earliest record of the theory of reincarnation, which comes from ancient Egypt, says that the soul is immortal; when the body perishes, the soul enters into another human body. Both early and present-day Hindus believe that the soul is immortal and inhabits one body after another in search of its true divine nature. Centuries before Christ, Buddha taught about the cycle of reincarnation—the great wheel of life and death. Like Hindus and Sikhs, Buddhists strive to be released from the death/rebirth cycle by attaining nirvana, or oneness with the Creator. In addition, the Essenes, an early Jewish sect; the medieval Christian Cathari, who flourished in France; and Islamic Sufis are also said to have embraced the idea of reincarnation.

The Greek philosopher Pythagoras, who lived some five centuries before Christ, not only wrote about this subject but also described his personal recollections of his various incarnations. His fellow philosopher Plato was also a believer. Napoleon claimed to have been the 8th-century Holy Roman emperor Charlemagne in a past life. The French philosopher Voltaire observed, "It's not more surprising to be born twice than once." The Spanish surrealist painter Salvador Dalí said that he believed he'd been the great Spanish mystic St. John of the Cross. And the 18th-century German writer and poet Johann Wolfgang von Goethe deeply embraced the idea of past lives as well: "I am certain that I've been here, as I am now, a thousand times before, and I hope to return a thousand times."

Many famous Americans, including Benjamin Franklin and Thomas Edison, also gave credence to reincarnation. George S. Patton, the famous American World War II general, believed that he'd been the Carthaginian general Hannibal in a previous life. Henry Ford, the father of modern assembly lines and mass production, was convinced that he'd lived before, too; and his most recent life had been as a soldier killed during the Battle of Gettysburg. Ralph Waldo Emerson, the American poet and essayist, subscribed to the notion of past lives.

Reincarnation is becoming more prevalent in Western culture as a viable personal belief system, because many people find that their spiritual needs aren't being met by current religions. Disillusioned individuals are turning instead to this philosophy, which answers questions such as "Why do we keep repeating the same negative patterns? Where do our recurring fears and phobias come from? Why do we feel an instant attraction to some people and places?" And more important, it helps to answer the question "What is our purpose here on Earth?" The concept of reincarnation allows us to understand the way in which we each weave our own destiny.

DAY 3

Soul Mates and Love Mates

Today we are going to look at one of the most important aspects of life that the philosophy of reincarnation addresses—relationships. Understanding and healing emotional difficulties that have their roots in past lives can help improve the quality of our present relationships. Our current partners, who are our karmic counterparts, give us the chance to complete unfinished tasks and help us release negative thoughts and emotions that intrude into this lifetime. Those with whom we have relationships that originated in a past life are called our "soul mates" or "love mates."

How many times have you caught a brief glimpse of someone across a crowded room and felt an instant rapport—an inner knowing that you've encountered a kindred spirit? In that brief moment, did you feel a yearning to rekindle those memories from the past and hold on to them for eternity? On the other hand, have you ever met someone and instantly felt uncomfortable, confused, or perhaps even angry for no apparent reason?

Such meetings are part of a complex web of intrigue that lies deep within our subconscious minds and dictates the tapestries of events that weave their way throughout our lifetimes. Our past-life relationships determine how we interact with those around us. They may also cause us to feel intense love or desire for an individual—or hatred, envy, or spite for another. As the soul memories are roused, relationships are rekindled. And almost everyone we connect with in this life is likely to have been involved in many of our past lives—perhaps as a brother, sister, parent, colleague, child, lover, or even an enemy.

The dynamics of our former-life situations are recreated in our present lives; and they may be passionate, romantic, and adventurous or even angry and vengeful. When we meet familiar souls in this current lifetime, it's to relive and rework the relationship. Those familiar eyes across a crowded room are often an inner reminder of the individuals whom we've chosen to interact with once more, and the encounter provides us with the opportunity to reexperience those karmic bonds.

The idea of a soul mate usually evokes images of Romeo and Juliet, Tristan and Isolde, or Katharine Hepburn and Spencer Tracy—individuals who found their perfect complement, becoming symbols of exquisite love that seem to transcend time and space. Although the term "soul mate" is commonly used to describe the one great love of your life, I prefer to call ideal partners "love mates." I believe that soul mates are actually *all* the individuals you've been with in past lives and even in other dimensions. This idea is based on the theory that you incarnate with the same individuals in each lifetime. You and your soul mates enter a lifetime together and are attracted to each other even from the far reaches of the world.

There's a tendency to think that our destined partners are the only ones to whom we feel an instant attraction; however, in my regression work, I've found that soul mates can also be the people we experience difficulties with in our present lives. In fact, such challenging individuals are often the ones we've had the most intimate past-life connections with.

When soul mates meet, there's usually an instant rapport, recognition, or even repulsion. If there was a sexual liaison in a past life, there will likely be a physical attraction in the present life—sometimes an intense and almost explosive one. Although soul mates don't always see eye to eye, there's usually a sense of familiarity in the relationship. They'll often have a communication beyond logical explanation and a deep attachment (either negative or positive) that is sometimes telepathic.

One of the greatest mysteries in the philosophy of reincarnation is the idea that every human being has a perfect partner. This person has been called a soul mate, dual mate, twin flame, and love mate— though I use the latter term to differentiate the one true love from all the soul mates or individuals who have been our companions or lovers in past lives. Researchers have stated that even in religions dating back to the Stone Age, one of the main reasons for leading a positive life was so that one could be reborn near his or her love mate in the next life. The writer and poet Goethe also wrote a book based on the medieval idea that couples were divinely united. *Die Wahlverwandtschaften*, which is usually translated as *Elective Affinities*, contends that every individual has a perfect mate waiting to be discovered.

A commonly-held theory regarding love mates is that we were originally androgynous beings—souls that were neither male nor female. Somewhere in time we were split in two and became either male or female energy but not necessarily two distinct bodies. These halves set forth into the Earth plane—a division of polarities growing and expanding, forever striving to reunite. The constant drive toward procreation is seen as a deep spiritual urge for that primal union and for the experience of oneness that occurred before the separation.

Those who adhere to this theory contend that there will be an increase in the search for and reunion with love mates in the coming years due to the increase in the vibratory rate of the planet. This accounts for the rise in relationships that transcend differences in race, age, gender, religion, and social standing.

Sometimes a love mate can be in the spirit world rather than in a physical body, offering assistance from the "other side." This can account for the feeling that a loving presence is watching over you. Soul mates can also be the same sex, although one will usually have the negative (feminine) polarity, while the other has the positive (masculine) polarity.

The degree to which you accept and love yourself plays an important role in your success in finding your love mate. If you feel unworthy while attempting to attract your destined partner, you'll start to think, *There must be something wrong with this person if he (or she) loves me.* You'll then subconsciously begin to find things wrong with the other person and push him or her away. Your love mate could even be the person you've been married to for the past 20 years, but you haven't been able to see the truth.

For many people, the philosophy of reincarnation, and of soul mates and love mates, provides an understanding of why we're here. It can give us insight into our current relationships and offer answers to some of life's seemingly unanswerable questions.

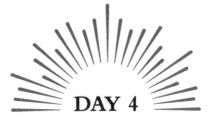

DAY 4

Karma, Destiny, and Free Will

Intrinsic to the understanding of reincarnation is a comprehension of karma, destiny, and free will, which are our topics for today. The principle that governs karma is "As ye sow, so shall ye reap." The fate we create for ourselves is a result of our judgments and actions in this life and in previous ones. Karma is the law of cause and effect—the universal ruling system that determines how we weave our destiny. It allows us to understand why one person is constantly dealt adversity, while another has a seemingly easy path.

In the past, karma was viewed as a kind of cosmic accounting system of debits and credits—a punitive and retributive law. Many once believed that all suffering was the result of previous wrongdoing— anything negative in one's life was caused by karma. However, this belief does a terrible injustice to anyone in an unfortunate situation.

The idea that karma is God's punitive system is now changing. The current opinion is much more compassionate and humane. There isn't an authority in the sky who decides what's right and wrong for each individual. Instead, inside each of us is an inner scale of justice monitoring our integrity. Our inner wisdom deems whether our actions are appropriate. The verdict isn't always what we consciously assume is right at the time, even if it's condoned by our religious or cultural beliefs. There are much deeper inner truths we adhere to, and sometimes they're beyond the rules of society.

I believe that we create not only our reality, but also our karma. So in your present life, you may subconsciously create difficult situations and find yourself being taken advantage of. I don't believe that this is cosmic punishment—it's a kind of inner balancing. When you feel deceived, you then have the opportunity to develop compassion for others who have had a similar experience. The extent to which you can accept yourself and all of your actions—and take responsibility for them (no matter what lifetime they occurred in)—is the extent to which you can step beyond karma. In other words, you've fulfilled your karma when you unconditionally forgive and accept yourself and others.

Forgiveness is the key to stepping off the karmic treadmill. (Remember, you don't need to forgive the act—because some are unforgivable—but it's important to forgive the individual or people who committed it.)

Karma can manifest itself in different ways. It can be demonstrated symbolically: People who in a past life were never willing to see the truth about themselves and the world around them might be born physically blind in a new life in order to learn how to perceive truth through intuition and feeling. I had a young client who couldn't swallow easily; through regression, we discovered that in a past life as a dancer she was forced into a situation that she couldn't swallow emotionally.

As life on our planet continues to speed up, we'll find ourselves balancing the karmic scales faster. I call this "instant karma." For example, if you judge someone for being inarticulate, the next day you may find yourself in a situation where your words seem jumbled and unclear. It's not a punishment, but rather your way of creating a circumstance that will allow you to be more understanding and less critical of others.

In any discussion of karma, it's important to bring up a viewpoint that many people hold: *I can't do anything about it. It's my karma.* No matter how difficult your life is, no matter what hardships you've endured, you're not stuck with your situation. You have the free will to change your circumstances or the way in which you view them. You're not bound to unalterable situations—the past, present, and future are malleable. You can change your karma and your resulting life circumstances.

I believe that each of us is born with a predestined future, and on the day we're born our date of death has already been decreed. However, as fervently as I believe in predestination, I also believe in free will. And I don't have difficulty holding these two seemingly divergent perspectives. Beyond linear time there's a changeable future and past, and it's possible to shift consciousness so that you can choose an entirely different timeline with a new subsequent past and future. In other words, you're not stuck with your past, and your future can be altered.

I've had some amazing experiences that make a solid case for predestination. When I was in southern Africa I met a very special Dutch woman who talked about having spent time in India. During her visits there, she heard of a remarkable place in the distant mountains where, generations ago, a famous astrologer once lived, and where his descendants had kept his records intact for hundreds of years. When the writing would become faded, they'd meticulously recopy the papers.

During this astrologer's life, whenever someone consulted him for a reading, not only did he compose a current chart, but he also drew up charts for their future lifetimes! He told his clients that if they came to retrieve their records in their future lives, they would be available for them.

At first I thought that this sounded almost too amazing to be true. Perhaps the legend was a ruse to make money. However, the Dutch woman told me that not only was no one ever charged for the charts, but visitors weren't even allowed to present flowers or other gifts.

She explained that she'd decided to travel to the astrologer's village with a friend. When she arrived, she told the villagers her place of birth and her birth date. They searched but weren't able to locate her chart—therefore, they concluded that she wasn't one of the individuals who'd had their charts prepared hundreds of years earlier. They did, however, find her friend's chart.

In her friend's present life, he had a very painful skin condition; and in his chart it said that during his incarnation in the 20th century, he would have a skin disease because he hadn't been kind to people with leprosy in a previous life. According to the chart, he must give generously to patients with leprosy in order to get rid of it. When he returned home from India, he donated to causes that were connected to this disease, and his skin condition completely cleared up. But when he eventually stopped giving to those charities, his skin problem returned.

I would have regarded this as no more than an interesting story, except that only a month later, when I was asked to take part in a BBC radio program in London, I heard a similar tale. At the end of the show, a soft-spoken Indian gentleman, a fellow guest who was a doctor and very famous sculptor, said, "There's something that I'd like to show you."

He pulled out a sheaf of faded papers covered in script that I assumed was ancient Sanskrit and proceeded to tell me that when he was 19 years old, he'd traveled with his father to a place where astrological records had been kept for hundreds of years. It sounded like the same place that the Dutch woman had described. After a long and arduous journey, the doctor and his father arrived on a rainy day, which was an unusual occurrence in that part of the world. They located the astrological charts for their present lives and found that both had indeed been clients of the famous astrologer hundreds of years before. The doctor told me that his chart stated that he'd come to claim his records when he was 19 years old, on a rainy day. His chart also correctly gave his name in his present life.

He went carefully through the chart with me (although I only had his word for what it said, as

I can't read Sanskrit) and showed me many more examples of where it had been accurate. I pass these stories along to you as they were shared with me. I found both individuals to be honest, trustworthy people. I believe them and their accounts.

DAY 5

Are Past Lives Real?

Today we are going to tackle a question I am often asked: Are past lives real or do we just make them up?

In order to heal and empower your present life, it's helpful to first know who and what you've been in previous incarnations. Past-life exploration is a highly effective method for traveling deep into the inner recesses of your mind to the place where memories of all your prior existences are stored. It can also be a direct path to the soul. As you uncover and heal old wounds from the past—and release self-limiting beliefs—you'll begin to understand your true purpose and place in the universe.

When you embark on a past-life regression, images and memories surface—sometimes in vivid detail. There are numerous documented cases of convincingly accurate details being recalled during past-life regressions, which are later validated through historical research. Participants of my seminars have also written to me and explained that they've investigated the lives that they saw during the group regression... and discovered that their visions were factual. However, most past lives haven't been recorded, so they've been lost forever, making it impossible to find written proof that your experiences before this lifetime were real.

You don't actually have to prove that your former lives are authentic—or even believe in reincarnation—to benefit from past-life therapy. When a person's life transforms—as a result of witnessing images that emerge during deep meditation—healing has occurred. It's not important if those images are "true" past lives or not; the significance lies in the advantages you receive while exploring their meaning. Even if the mental pictures that come to the surface aren't past-life memories but are simply symbols from your subconscious, they deserve to be probed. They're legitimate expressions from your inner being, which can greatly increase the quality of your life.

When they discover a previous incarnation, participants in my past-life seminars sometimes say, "Am I just making this up?" I tell them to stop worrying about whether the images they see are real or not. The value lies in the results they achieve in their lives based on what they've learned from the regression—it's not about wondering if they're recalling a fantasy lifetime.

Although many of the memories you experience will be factual, proving their validity is a lot less important than the profound growth that can occur in your life just by viewing them. And on a spiritual level, of course you're making it up. You're always "making it up," no matter what you're experiencing, because the circumstances of your life come from the creative force within you. In no small way—in every moment—you're imagining and manifesting your life. So to remember your past lives, just let go and be willing to "make it up."

In our culture we're told to dismiss anything that doesn't fit within the normal consensus of reality. The reluctance to accept past-life memories may have its roots in our collective childhood, in which imagination was demeaned and relegated to the inconsequential world of make-believe. When children talk about an invisible friend or when someone sees a ghost or an angel, these individuals are told to ignore it, because it's "just their imagination." When people say, "Oh, that's just her imagination," and reduce its value in such a pejorative way, it's truly a desecration of one of our most sacred faculties—the ability to tap into our intuitive and visionary capacity.

Our imagination is one of the most powerful spiritual tools that we possess, for it's an entrance into other worlds and the pathway used by ancient seers to pierce into other dimensions and travel through time and space. Mystics and prophets also rely on it to traverse the subtle inner realm and access universal truths. It's a sacred ability of all human beings, so I invite you to awaken your creative spark and explore what and who you've been. Allow your imagination free rein without constantly questioning the images, and you'll begin to receive more accurate information regarding your previous lives. Remember that this faculty is a hallowed doorway to your far past.

Past-life journeys can sometimes provide the answers that traditional medicine or therapy can't. Of course there may be many contributing reasons for our problems—it can be all too easy to blame current difficulties on past-life behavior or actions. Nevertheless, exploration into earlier lives has proven to be incredibly powerful in many situations where other methods have failed. By knowing who we've been in previous lives, we can better understand our place and mission in the present. Life isn't a one-time affair, nor is it a series of meaningless experiences strung together. A journey backward in time will assist the process of gradually realizing our full potential as conscious, loving beings.

DAY 6

How to Discover Who You Were

Discovering who you were in a past life can be easy and fun! There are a number of methods you can employ, and over the next several days you'll learn how to uncover amazing evidence of your previous lives. By asking yourself pertinent questions you will explore various areas of your present life, which will help you open the door into your previous incarnations; in addition, the questions are specifically designed as a kind of touchstone to activate memories, emotions, and images from long ago. In almost mystical ways, each question acts as a key to unlock your past.

When you examine the present, you can pick up hundreds of clues that can help you glean information from the past. This is a powerful way to open the door for spontaneous past-life recall, without requiring you to go into an altered state of consciousness. You might even think of yourself as a past-life detective as you amass clues from your affinities and experiences in your current life.

Try writing each of the topics we cover in the following chapters at the top of a separate sheet of paper in a special notebook—what I call your Past-life Detective Journal. As you answer the questions below each subject heading, write down all the "clues" that you can gather. You may want to place the completed sheets side by side so that a larger picture can begin to form.

It can be helpful to center yourself before answering each question. If a seemingly unrelated thought or memory arises as you do the exercise, write it down. Pay attention to all of your reactions; sometimes a small clue can open a big door.

Go through the following chapters in a thoughtful manner. Proceed slowly, allowing yourself to reflect, breathe, and contemplate. Ask yourself, *If the answer to this question opened a portal to another time period, where would I be... and who would I have been?* The more time and energy you allow, the more likely you are to truly discover who you were.

Notice the feelings that each question elicits. As you embark on this comprehensive journey, stay in touch with any emotions or spontaneous physical sensations that begin to emerge. Again, I suggest you write down your answers. You'll gain clearer and more accurate insights the more thorough you are in accessing your responses.

When I did this exercise, I saw that I had amassed evidence indicating a past life in Japan. I've always loved the simple lines of traditional Japanese architecture. In my current life, not only did I live for more than two years in a Japanese Buddhist monastery, but I also studied this culture while I was attending the University of Hawaii. Moreover, I've learned about the Japanese tea ceremony and ikebana (flower arranging) and trained in the healing systems of Reiki and shiatsu. In addition, my favorite restaurants have always been Japanese! And to top it off, there was a period in my life when I saw every samurai movie that was available—at that time, I held Toshiro Mifune in the same regard as people hold famous actors today. Looking at these clues as a reincarnation detective, it makes sense that I had a past life in the Far East.

As you create your lists, pay special attention to your emotional responses toward each topic. For example, under "Clues from Your Relationships," as well as considering your relationships with fellow humans, be sure to do the exercise about animals, too. I know a man who has a very close attachment to horses. He was a Mongolian in a past life and during that time, he loved his horse even more than his wife. In the chapter "Clues from Your Name and Your Characteristics," examine any personal quirks that you may have. I met a woman who rubs her throat whenever she feels stress. She discovered that in a previous life she'd been stabbed in the throat; and in her current life, any kind of stress subconsciously activates her past-life memory.

Patterns will start to emerge as you gather your clues. You may ask yourself, *How will I know if I'm accurate? How can I distinguish between simple fascination and a stirring of deep, inner knowing?* A good indication is usually your emotional response. If it feels right, it probably is. If you're unsure, meditate upon the ideas that are beginning to form from your insights. Even if you're not completely clear, sooner or later your subconscious will show you the path to greater understanding. In particular, watch your dreams after you've finished answering the questions.

Past-life memories often begin to unfold during the nighttime hours.

Once you've answered all the questions and compiled lists of clues, study this information and you'll be able to begin piecing together the puzzle, forming a picture of some of your past-life scenarios. It's not uncommon for people to have spontaneous former-life memories. Trust in the process. These kinds of memories arise when the time is right for you to process and heal them. Have faith that the time is right. Notice—and write down—any similarity or connection between these recollections and your current life.

Remember that no single factor can provide all the answers, but if you gather them together, you can begin to solve the puzzle of who you might have been in previous incarnations.

DAY 7

Clues from Your Childhood

Today you will start your past-life detective work with a look at your childhood. As a child, you didn't have the strong filters most adults later develop that block out past-life memories; therefore, careful examination of your childhood preferences, inclinations, and the games you enjoyed when you were little can often reveal significant evidence about who you were.

Asking family members what you were like as a child can be helpful. The younger the child, the more potent past-life memories usually are. My grandmother told me that when I was three, I'd get very irritated with her because she didn't remember our previous life together. She said that I'd plaintively ask again and again, "Don't you remember when we were sisters?"

When my daughter, Meadow, was three, she used to talk about her servants. I found this rather curious, considering that we maintained a casual lifestyle and often ate our meals seated on the floor. (This could probably be traced to my Native American life, sitting and eating by the fire.) However, even as a three-year-old, Meadow insisted on sitting at the table and would place numerous spoons, forks, and knives neatly next to her plate, as if in a formal dinner setting. Then she'd ask me to arrange the food on her plate into a beautiful presentation. This ritual was very important to her and was completely different from our brown-rice-with-vegetables lifestyle.

She'd also request that I place her clothes on the bed. She'd plead, "My servants used to lay my clothes out for me. I don't know how to dress myself." When her friends came over, Meadow would organize genteel games along with elaborate tea parties. One day they went outside to play, and I encouraged her to join them. She responded gravely, "I'm not allowed to play outdoors with other children. I must not soil my clothes." The pain and sadness of a lonely royal had seemingly filtered down into her childhood games.

Children's attitudes can often be attributed to their environment or upbringing, but I don't think this is the case for Meadow, as my husband and I are relaxed and informal. Meadow continues to be quite the lady; however, I can't help but think that she chose us as parents in order to balance a past life that was extremely traditional and rigid.

One of my friends told me that one day, many years ago, she was driving in her car with her four-year-old daughter and when they drove over a bridge, the little girl casually said, "These are the killing waters."

Shocked, my friend asked her daughter what she meant, and she proceeded to tell her mom that she had drowned in the water below when she and her "other brother" were swimming, and her "other mother" was very sad. My friend, who had no interest in reincarnation at the time, researched local papers and discovered that more than 30 years earlier, a brother and sister had been swimming at that exact spot… and the young girl had drowned. (As my friend's daughter grew older, she lost all memories of this event.)

While the most common childhood games are the result of programming by society (for example, a young girl is given a baby doll and is told that she is its mother), sometimes, playtime activities are a residue of memories from earlier lives.

When I was six, I used to explore the woods by our house and would spend hours alone picking small bits of different plants and tasting them. I'd bring a bunch of my selections home, let them dry, and then attempt to grind the dried plants into powder.

I called my concoctions "medicine" and would try to get my friends to take some if they weren't feeling well. I now believe that this activity was based on my memories as a Blackfoot Indian, gathering medicinal herbs for my tribe.

A skeptic might say this behavior could have been the result of being influenced by stories I'd heard or information that I'd subconsciously absorbed from my mom or dad. But my parents never used herbs and neither did my Cherokee grandparents. Why would a six-year-old fixate on one particular activity to the exclusion of all others? There can be many reasons, and one answer is that it can be traced to a previous life.

And how does a skeptical individual explain a child who's a master musician even though his or her parents aren't musically talented? Although it's impossible to prove beyond a doubt that reincarnation occurs, it's enormously valuable to observe childhood games, for they often hold important keys to understanding past lives.

Now list every idiosyncrasy that was unique to you as a child and think about what kind of previous life might have been responsible for that personal trait.

Exercise:
Examining Clues from Your Childhood Preferences, Inclinations, and Games

Ask yourself the following questions and jot down the answers in your Past-life Detective Journal.

- What consistent attitudes did you have about life as a youth? When given choices, did you have any strong preferences?

- Did your family members tell you about anything unusual you did? Did you have any habits or predilections that were uncommon for a child of your age?

- What were the types of games you played as a child? List them. Were any of these unusual for someone of your age? What did you like to wear for costume parties?

- As you go through your list, were there any activities that consistently brought up particular emotions? Did your friends play any games that made you feel uncomfortable?

- When you were playing make-believe, what did you envision?

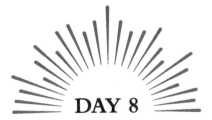

DAY 8

Clues from Your Tastes

Valuable clues to your past lives can often be found in your tastes, which is our topic for today. Your preferred clothing, architecture, home furnishings, foods, smells, music, books, and movies can all be fruitful areas for you to explore.

Clothing, Architecture, and Home Furnishings

Let's start with clothing you're drawn to (or that you detest). For example, are you attracted to boho, peasant, or military fashions? Do you enjoy wearing long dresses or dinner jackets, or do you loathe formal wear and just like to feel comfortable? Are there certain types of hats that you've worn regularly? A French man I knew who always wore a cowboy hat found that he was once a cowboy in the 19th-century Wild West. The colors of clothing may also have past-life significance. For example, I knew a woman who always appeared in saffron-yellow garments—it was more or less her trademark. During a regression, she recalled being a Hindu monk in India, wearing saffron-colored robes daily.

As you examine your clothing preferences, be aware of any styles that you're drawn to from particular cultures or time periods. Also think about the kinds of outfits you like to wear to costume parties.

Next let's look at the architectural styles that you admire. Are you fascinated by Tudor, Georgian, or Victorian designs; or are you interested in structures such as cabins, tepees, yurts, cliff dwellings, or perhaps even castles and Greek temples?

Your home furnishings are another kind of clue into your past. Does your home resemble a cottage in England? Perhaps you once lived in the English countryside. Another thing to examine is your relationship to your home. Do you tend to move often? This can indicate a prior experience of living a nomadic lifestyle. Do you want to stay in one house forever? This points to a past life where you were born and lived your entire life in one residence. Alternatively, this could also signify a previous incarnation as someone who always longed to have a permanent home.

Take a moment to look around your home, and observe your surroundings objectively. Be aware of any furnishings from a particular era or geographical location. Draw a picture of your perfect home— inside and out—and notice what emotions and images arise as you do so.

Exercise:
Analyzing Your Taste in Clothing,
Architecture, and Home Furnishings

Ask yourself the following questions and jot down the answers in your Past-life Detective Journal.

- What styles of clothing do you really like and dislike? What is your favorite outfit and why?

- What footwear do you like most? Be specific.

- What is your favorite architectural style? What is your least favorite? Why?

- What type of furnishings do you like or strongly dislike? What colors are predominant in your home?

- Have you moved around a lot in your life, or do you have a tendency to stay in one place?

Food Preferences, Eating Habits, Scents, and Smells

Your childhood associations around eating and food preparation can often be indicative of past lives, and sometimes the types of food that you're attracted to as an adult can offer previous-life clues. If asked to pick what you enjoy the most, would you choose Indian, Chinese, Thai, Japanese, French, Italian, Greek, African, Spanish, Mexican, English, Scandinavian, German, Russian, Vietnamese, Hungarian, or some other cuisine? What cooking style or ingredients do you prefer? For example, if you really love pineapples and papayas, this might indicate that you once lived in a tropical climate.

How you consume your meals can also offer important clues. Do you eat like a peasant? King? Monk? Samurai? List your favorite and least favorite types of food. Notice what emotions each food elicits in you. Stand in your kitchen and notice how you feel when you're in there or as you're preparing a meal.

Although we ascribe great importance to the way something tastes, the way it smells can have an even more powerful effect on our emotions than any of our other senses. A scent can instantly transport you to another time in this life or in history. Almost all smells have subconscious memories associated with them. Notice the powerful reactions—positive and negative—that you've had to certain odors you've encountered in your life. Then imagine what kind of experience someone might have had in order to strongly like or dislike that particular scent.

Exercise: Exploring Your Food Preferences, Eating Habits, Scents, and Smells

Ask yourself the following questions and jot down the answers in your Past-life Detective Journal.

- As a child, what foods did you love and hate? Was there any particular way that you used to enjoy eating your meals?

- How do you consume your food? Do you eat quickly, almost as if it were your last meal (like someone who normally doesn't have much to eat), or do you eat in an elegant and refined manner (like someone who has the luxury of picking at their food)?

- Are there any foods that always upset your stomach? Are there any that bring on an emotional response within you—either positive or negative?

- What scents do you love or hate? Have you ever had an immediate and powerful emotional reaction to an odor but didn't know why?

- Imagine gently breathing in each of the following aromas and see if any spontaneous memories arise (after each one, I've listed where it was popular in past times): frankincense or myrrh (Middle East); sandalwood (India); eucalyptus (Australia); lemon (Italy); juniper (Tibet); lavender (France); sage (North America); and rose (England).

Music, Books, Films, and TV

A song or musical score has the ability to transport us back to the time when we first heard it. A forgotten memory can be conjured simply by listening to a piece that was being played during the event. Just as music can help us evoke memories from this life, it can also spur remembrances of past lives.

When you listen to music, is there a certain kind that creates images in your mind? Imagine that you're traveling the world and hearing the rhythms and songs from every country and time period. Is there a particular era or area that you really like or dislike?

Searching for clues to your past lives can be as easy as reading travel guides and watching films situated in other countries or time periods to observe your reactions to various scenes and images. Read about different cultures in an encyclopedia (or online) and note which ones you find most interesting. Look at pictures of various environments and notice how they affect you.

Make a list of times when you've read a book or watched a film or TV show and felt instantly transported into a realm that seemed real and familiar to you. In addition, write down any intensely strong emotions that surprised you while you were reading or watching a movie or TV. Your lists are good starting points for past-life exploration.

Exercise:
Delving into Your Taste in Music, Books, Films, and TV

Ask yourself the following questions and jot down the answers in your Past-life Detective Journal.

* As a child, was there a specific kind of music that you liked or disliked? What's your favorite type of music now? Is there a genre that always makes you happy or sad, or particularly emotional?

- Have you ever learned to play a musical instrument? Do you still play it? Were you able to learn it easily—that is, did it seem familiar to you?

- As a child, was there a particular book that fascinated you or one that you read over and over? What was it about the story that made such an impression on you?

- What is your favorite book? Why? What kind of stories do you like to read? Do you have a favorite writer?

- What types of movies or TV series do you like or dislike, and why? Westerns? War movies? Shows about families? Action films? Medical dramas? Historical epics? Cop shows? Love stories? And so on.

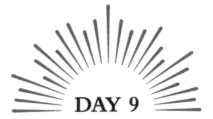

DAY 9

Clues from Your Name and Your Characteristics

Today we are going to look at how our names, personality traits, heritage, talents, abilities, occupations and hobbies all reveal information relating to our previous incarnations.

Names, Personality Traits, and Heritage

The name that you currently possess isn't an accident. In addition to providing you with the vibration and energy that you need for your current life, there are often past-life correlations with it.

If you've been named after a family member, there's almost always a karmic connection with that individual. Rose had been named after her great-grandmother. Although she'd never met her, when she researched their family tree, she found remarkable similarities between them. The similarities were so strong that the younger Rose became convinced that she'd been her great-grandmother in her former life.

Be sure not to overlook the nicknames that either you take on yourself or that others give you. A woman named Merry was called "Medici" for her entire life, for no obvious reason that anyone could remember. However, during a regression she uncovered a life in Italy as part of the powerful Medici family.

More details about your past lives can be found by studying the mannerisms, personality quirks, and behaviors that make you unique. Of course many of these characteristics can be traced to events and influences in your present life, but the traits that are completely out of keeping with your upbringing can be explained by exploring past lives. It's also not uncommon, as a karmic balancing, to undergo a complete personality reversal.

Sometimes habitual behaviors can be explained in terms of reincarnation. Fran had a peculiar trait of bowing to everyone she met. Although this isn't unusual behavior for someone who had a previous life in Asia, it was considered strange in her present life.

Your personality wasn't just formed upon birth; it's the outcome of a long line of incarnations. Jot down the adjectives that best describe you. Look at this list and imagine that someone in history had these same qualities; think about where this person might have lived and what might have been their occupation.

There's often a correlation between a person's cultural and/or racial heritage and the types of past lives he or she has experienced. This link isn't always evident, and to date there's been very little research into this phenomenon.

You may find that you've shared a life with one or more of your ancestors or that you actually have been one of your own ancestors. Deborah was surprised when, during a regression, she realized that she'd been her great-aunt Esther. Upon further research, she was even more astounded to discover an incredible number of similarities in their lives. For example, each year on her birthday, Deborah always performed a secret ceremony early in the morning. Later in her life, Deborah was given Esther's diary and read her great-aunt's entries that recounted doing the exact same thing!

It's also common to have a number of past lives in the same heritage. So if you're of Scottish ancestry, you might have had a number of Scottish lifetimes; if you're of African descent, you might have had a number of African lifetimes. (I'm not sure if we actually have more lives in a particular heritage or if they're just easier to "remember" because they're somehow familiar to us.)

If others constantly assume that you're a different heritage than what you think you are, this can also be a past-life clue. If you don't know much about your ancestry, you may want to do some research to become more familiar with your roots. Many people find that this dovetails very well with their own past-life exploration.

Exercise:
Examining Your Name, Personality Traits, and Heritage

Ask yourself the following questions and jot down the answers in your Past-life Detective Journal.

- What's the meaning of your name? What nationality is your name? Are you named after someone—a family member, perhaps? What do you know about that person?

- When you were growing up, did you have any nicknames? Do you have a name that you go by that isn't your legal name? What's the significance of that name, and what does it mean to you?

- How would others describe your personality? How would you describe it? Do you have any personality quirks or unusual mannerisms?

- Do you have any habitual behaviors but aren't quite sure why or how they started? List them. If a historical play were performed that starred someone who exhibited these same characteristics, who and what might that person be?

- What is your heritage? Are you closely aligned with any of your ancestors, or are there any whom you identify with? Do you feel attracted to any cultures that are also a part of your heritage?

Talents, Abilities, Occupations, and Hobbies

Many of the abilities that come to you spontaneously and easily can be attributed to past lives. Perhaps child prodigies—such as Mozart—acquire their abilities from previous lives. Examining your natural talents might offer additional clues as to who you once were.

One Saturday morning my daughter, Meadow, announced that she wanted to go ice-skating. My husband, David, is usually very slow to move in the morning, so I was astounded when he immediately agreed—especially since he'd never skated in his life.

My daughter had roller-skated before but had never ice-skated, and she quickly plopped down onto the ice. I'd skated as a child, but I was rusty and shaky. So, we were amazed when David, the non-skater, sailed past us effortlessly with the most smooth, graceful movements. He glided around us in circles. He skated backward. He completed wondrous spins and turns. Astonishing!

Despite eventually pulling a muscle in his knee, David seemed to know exactly how to skate. Previously he'd recalled a life as a city official in Holland, and he had often skated on frozen canals and ponds. I believe that those distant memories of Holland had filtered through from his past.

Talents from our past lives often emerge during our childhood years… and then sometimes they recede as we enter adulthood. Think about any unusual talents you possessed as a child or whether you feel a natural pull toward any particular skills. List these abilities and imagine that if there was a past life associated with each one of these talents, what would that life have been like?

The occupations we're drawn to are usually the same as, or have similar features to, the ones we undertook in past lives. This seems to be especially true of vocations in early life. For example, one man whom I regressed had been a piano maker in Germany. In his current life, he learned to play that instrument as he was growing up, and in his twenties he became a carpenter. Both of these skills were connected to his previous life. Now he is neither a pianist nor a carpenter—he's an artist. I believe that he'd completed the karma from his prior German life, so he's no longer involved in the same occupations or hobbies.

Your career can often indicate skills that you possessed in one or more of your previous incarnations. Sometimes your occupation is a continuing aspect of an earlier one; or as a way to balance karma, your current job could be a reversal of those that you had in past lives.

Exercise:
Exploring Your Talents, Abilities, Occupations, and Hobbies

Ask yourself the following questions and jot down the answers in your Past-life Detective Journal.

- In what particular area of your life do you naturally excel? What abilities do you admire or dislike in others?

- Have you ever surprised yourself by innately knowing how to do something? What was it? Have you ever created something—or truly excelled at something–that evoked strong and familiar emotions?

- When you were a child, what did you want to be when you grew up? Did you follow your childhood passion? Were there aspects of your youthful desires that you pursued?

- What is your present career? Do you like it? Is it easy or difficult for you?

- Do you have any hobbies? If you could pursue any hobby, without expense or time as a consideration, what would you enjoy doing? Why?

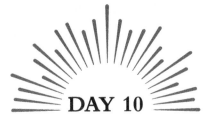

DAY 10

Clues from Your Body and Your Health

It's not uncommon for certain physical features and health challenges to reemerge lifetime after lifetime, so these are our topics for today.

Body Type and Health Issues

Although we have different body types in our various lives, sometimes there are aspects that carry over from a previous lifetime. Usually this only occurs if there's a blockage or emotional response that wasn't cleared from an earlier life, but sometimes it happens because we strongly identify with a characteristic.

Ronald was born with one arm slightly deformed. Surprisingly, when I asked him how it made him feel, he said that he felt like a coward. When I regressed him back in time, he relived a life as a Japanese warrior who was no longer allowed to fight after sustaining serious injury. This made him feel inferior and even weak for not fighting alongside his compatriots. Healing that lifetime didn't change the status of his arm, but he no longer viewed himself as a coward.

An incident that's similar to a past-life event can activate an unaccounted pain or injury that originated in the far past. There can also be residual memories of health issues that will filter into the present and manifest in your current body. For example, heart problems (or a broken heart) in a past life can resurface as heart disease in a current life. However, health problems will only be repeated if there were unresolved issues of this kind during the past-life experience.

Additionally, a disease or illness that you had at a particular age in your past life can emerge at the same age in your present life. This will only happen if there are unresolved emotional issues that accompanied this event. Dakota developed a terrible rash that covered her body when she was 25 years old. The onset was sudden and dramatic, and it even erupted into severe blisters. In a regression, she saw a past life in which she'd been 25 years old and had been burned at the stake for being a witch.

Some present-day health concerns are a symbolic manifestation of a past-life trauma. For example, throat problems can come from an incarnation in which you were hanged, strangled, or killed for speaking your truth, while severe headaches could be due to massive head wounds or battle injuries.

Simply focusing intently on the part of your body that's chronically out of balance can often ignite images from the past.

Exercise: Analyzing Your Body and Health Issues

Ask yourself the following questions and jot down the answers in your Past-life Detective Journal.

- What is your body type? Is it slender, frail, muscular, athletic, portly, or small? Do you possess any unusual physical features? Were you born with them, or did they develop later in life?

- Do you feel comfortable in your skin? Or does your body not fit who you feel you truly are?

- Did you have any recurring health issues during childhood? What was your emotional response to health concerns when you were a child? Do you have any physical disabilities?

- Have you always believed that you'd live a long life? Why? Alternatively, have you ever thought that your life would be short? Why?

- Are you committed to alternative-health remedies or to allopathic medicine? If you seek holistic methods, do you respond well to Chinese herbs and acupuncture, Western herbs, Ayurvedic massage, hydrotherapy, cleansing steams, colonics, or crystal therapy? (Often the type of treatment that works the best for you—or the worst—is a reflection of a past-life remedy.)

Scars, Birthmarks, Tattoos, Injuries, and Diseases

There's a definite correlation between scars, birthmarks, and tattoos that you may have in this life and what has occurred in your past lives. In a regression, a woman vividly remembered having been shot in the forehead in another life. Interestingly enough, this woman found an unusual, small indentation beneath her hairline that looked as if a small bullet had penetrated there.

Even birthmarks can carry clues to past lives. I suggest that you examine your birthmarks and ask yourself what might have made those specific kinds of marks; then pay attention to any images or feelings that well up from within you.

Tattoos can also give past-life hints. Over a number of years, Marie had had Celtic symbols tattooed on various parts of her body and was comforted when she discovered a previous life in Ireland as a blacksmith.

Look over your body and write down any scars, birthmarks, and tattoos that you have. Draw an outline of your body and indicate exactly where they are—note even the smallest ones. Pay particular attention to areas that have been scarred several times in the exact same places. A simple guided meditation into the area of a recurrent scar (or birthmark) can often reveal past-life memories.

Not only are the injuries and diseases that you've endured often indicative of past-life experiences, but the emotions that have accompanied them are also very telling. Sue-Ann became unusually despondent and even fatalistic every time she caught a cold. She only figured out why when she experienced a past life in Portugal in which a summer cold had quickly led to pneumonia and then to her death.

To delve even deeper into your previous lives, whenever you're hurt, imagine that you're actually becoming very tiny and traveling into the injury or wound. Then allow images and memories to rise to the surface. The closer to the time of the injury, the easier it is to discover your incarnation.

The mishaps that your body has encountered aren't usually an accident. List every injury, disease, and surgery that you've ever had. Then write down the emotions that each one brings up for you. Notice if there is any similarity in the feelings that arise.

Exercise: Examining Your Scars, Birthmarks, Tattoos, Injuries, Diseases, and Surgeries

Ask yourself the following questions and jot down the answers in your Past-life Detective Journal.

- How old were you were when you obtained your scars? How did you get them? Do you have any emotions associated with them?

- If you have a birthmark, where is it on your body? Does its shape resemble anything? If you have tattoos, are they from any particular culture or specific era?

- Have you had any recurring injuries in a particular place on your body? If there was a soul drama that might account for that specific injury, what might it be?

- Have you had any unusual diseases or illnesses? What part of your body was affected?

- What kinds of surgeries have you had? Why? Did the medical procedure heal the condition? What else was occurring in your life at the time?

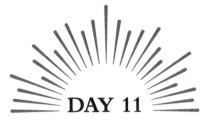

DAY 11

Clues from Your Relationships

Today we are considering relationships because, perhaps more than any other clues, the dynamics of our relationships can offer powerful insights into who we were in our past lives.

Human Relationships

We tend to subconsciously and symbolically recreate events from our far past, especially from those experiences that were never resolved. Every reenactment is a way to heal those unsettled situations. For example, when Moses and John were growing up, they were next-door neighbors. They were friends but Moses always resented John, and for some reason John put up with it. One summer they went on a canoe trip together. As they paddled, their canoe overturned and Moses was caught in the current. John, at great effort—and almost at the expense of his own life—was able to rescue Moses.

From that point their relationship almost magically transformed, and Moses no longer resented his friend. John later discovered that in a past life, they'd both been native South Americans. On a canoe trip during that lifetime, Moses had fallen out of the boat but John didn't try to save him. Moses had drowned, which caused the lingering resentment in the present time. Reliving the original event shifted the dynamics between them.

Often the way you feel about someone is a reflection of a past connection. For instance, whenever Jill talked about her friend Sandy, she called her "my sister." Jill discovered that in a previous life, Sandy had been her younger sister. This explained why she felt the need to protect and support Sandy in her current life.

Also, just because someone seems to be your enemy in this life, it doesn't necessarily mean that there's a negative past life. In some cases, a very loving soul mate will incarnate at your request to be a worthy opponent; as a result, you are able to gain strength, clarity, and wisdom as you overcome your adversary. In other words, this individual came in order to help you grow. By carefully examining all your relationships, and especially the recurring patterns, you can begin to understand the dynamics of your past.

Every one of your important relationships is with someone you've known before. Additionally, the patterns that occur with partners in your current life have their source in your past. Make a list of every significant relationship that you've had in your life— both ones that you deem positive and negative. Then after each entry, write a few words that describe the relationship's dynamics and how it feels or felt at the time. For example, you might write "feels like fellow warriors," or "feels like mother and son." Notice any past-life images that begin to emerge.

Exercise: Exploring Your Human Relationships

Ask yourself the following questions and jot down the answers in your Past-life Detective Journal.

- As a child, who was most important to you? Whom did you feel safe with? Was there anyone you felt unsafe around? Who loved you and whom did you love?

- What was the main way that you related to people as a child? Were you shy or aloof, or did you want to be the life of the party? Did you desire to be lord of the manor? Were you always trying to make everyone happy?

- As an adult, what patterns—regarding your relationships—seem to recur? Do you constantly attend to the needs of others, even to the detriment of your own needs? Do you sabotage relationships? Are you taken advantage of frequently, or do you take advantage of others?

- Who have been your best friends? When you met them, did you feel an instant bond? Who have been your enemies? When you first came into contact with these individuals, did you immediately have feelings of like or dislike toward them?

- Do you feel close to your family, or have you felt that you've never quite belonged? Whom do you feel most connected to—either in a negative and positive way—and which family member do you feel the most detached from?

Relationships with Animals and Pets

Do you feel a kinship with certain kinds of animals? When you're around these beings, do you feel that you're able to communicate with them? This type of experience may be related to a past life in which you had extensive contact with a particular kind of animal. Perhaps you were a horse trainer or a farmer.

Or maybe at some point, your only friend was a pet. There are accounts of prisoners who formed bonds with rats in their cells and even saved portions of their meager rations to feed their little friends. These acts of kindness, along with gratitude for the animals, kept these individuals from going insane.

To the ancient Egyptians, cats represented gods. Relics of that time are filled with regal pictures of cats acting out the civilization's most important myths. In fact, cats were so honored that many of them were embalmed along with their owners when they died. If you've had a lifelong affinity for cats, you might have had a life in ancient Egypt.

Sometimes an animal that unreasonably frightens you can be an important sign. For example, Donald was terrified of alligators. He was so frightened that he refused to swim in his pool at night because of his intense fear—even though there were no alligators in New Mexico where he lived. It was only when he healed a past life—in which he'd been dragged into the water and mauled by a crocodile—that he could finally enjoy nighttime swims in his pool without fear.

Carefully analyzing the types of animals you're drawn to—as well as those you're afraid of—can offer remarkable clues to your past. Make a list of all the animals you've been attached to, fascinated with, or terrified of in your life. After each entry, imagine a past-life scenario that includes the animal and your associated emotions. Write it all down.

Exercise: Delving into Your Relationships with Animals and Pets

Ask yourself the following questions and jot down the answers in your Past-life Detective Journal.

- What animals do you love or admire? Which ones do you dislike?

- If you had to be an animal, which kind would you like to be?

- Do you have any paintings, statues, or figurines of a certain animal in your home?

- Do you have collections of one particular kind of animal? Why? What associations do you have with that species?

- Have you discovered your totem animal? What is it? In what part of the world or historical time-period were these animals revered?

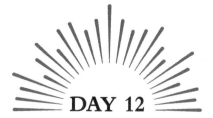

DAY 12

Clues from Places, Events, Cultures, and Déjà Vu

Today we are going to consider how locations, climates, cultures, time periods, historical events, and even the feeling of déjà vu can help us discover more about our previous incarnations.

Geographical Locations and Climates

An excellent exercise to activate past-life memories is to imagine yourself in a variety of terrains. Immerse all of your senses... sights, sounds, scents, textures, and so on, as you imagine each environment. What feeling does each locale evoke within you? Be open to every nuance of your experience, as this will often trigger memories from your far past. When Peggy tried this exercise, she found that every time she imagined being surrounded by snowcapped mountains, she felt immensely happy. She discovered that this was consistent with a previous life in which she'd owned goats and resided in the mountains of Switzerland.

Although you might think that almost everyone would prefer a temperate climate, it's surprising how much variety there is in people's weather preferences. A strong emotional response to specific conditions often has its source in a past life. For example, Samuel, who lived in a farming community in Iowa, loved steamy hot climates. Even as a child, he asked his mom to paint a jungle scene in his bedroom. In his past-life regression, he recalled living in a humid rain forest—a lush jungle where monkeys flew effortlessly through the treetops.

If you love extreme, arid heat, perhaps you once lived in a desert; or if you prefer the clean, crisp coolness of wintertime, you may have enjoyed a past life in a land of snow and ice. Imagine yourself in different climates and note the emotional responses you have to each.

Exercise: Analyzing Geographical Locations and Climates

Ask yourself the following questions and jot down the answers in your Past-life Detective Journal.

- What countries have you always wanted to visit? Where have you never wanted to go? If you could vacation anywhere in the world, where would you go and why?

- What kind of terrain makes you feel at your best— and where do you feel the worst? Is it in the desert, plains, savanna, mountains, rain forest, pine forest, at the beach or by a lake? Is it in a meadow or by rolling hills, valleys, or canyons?

- Which do you prefer: cities, towns, villages, farms, ranches, or the countryside?

- What's your favorite type of climate? What countries have the kind of climate that you like (or dislike) the most? (The first names that pop into your mind may be a clue.)

- Do you prefer being outside or indoors? What kind of weather makes you feel happy? Sad? Depressed? Content? Creative?

Cultures, Time Periods, Historical Events, and Déjà Vu

Carefully examining the cultures that you're interested in can offer you a pathway back into your past. Jason loved the ancient Egyptian civilization. Even as a child, his most prized possession was an ankh that his uncle brought him from a vacation to Egypt. His interest grew as a teen, and as an adult, Jason visited museum exhibits of Egyptian artifacts. He wasn't surprised when he discovered a past life in Egypt.

There's often a correlation between the cultures that fascinate you and your past incarnations. For example, someone who's deeply interested in Native Americans or the Aztec civilization may find that he or she has experienced a previous life in that society. Also notice the ethnic designs that appeal or feel familiar to you. Look at symbols from various peoples such as Celtic, Egyptian, Maori, Native American, African, Chinese, Japanese, Indian, Viking, Roman, and Middle Eastern.

A historical event or time period that you feel strongly drawn to is most likely an indication of a past life, so it's valuable to examine this interest. My father didn't believe in reincarnation; however, he wasn't so sure after he explored our Scottish roots and ancestry. He told me about his experience standing on a high moor and suddenly "seeing" a battle and feeling that he absolutely knew every nuance of it as it unfolded before his eyes. This event was startling to him, and my dad felt as if he'd been there long ago.

Examine periods in history that have interested you in your present life. Cast your mind back to your school days—was there a particular era that appealed to you then, such as the Stone Age, the Bronze Age, the ancient rule of the pharaohs, the Middle Ages, the Renaissance, or the Industrial Revolution? Are there historical events that captivate you now?

Briefly consult any world-history reference work to see if there's a certain epoch that stands out in your mind; however, remember that many books of this genre ignore native cultures, so you'll have to look in anthropology books for this type of information.

The phenomenon of déjà vu can make you feel as if you are reliving a moment in your own history. However, psychologists say that déjà vu occurs when the scene that you're observing becomes available to your conscious mind a split second before you're consciously aware of it. You sense that you've seen it or been there before because you have—a fraction of a second earlier. However, I've found a direct correlation between déjà vu and past lives and believe that these events are very important in exploring reincarnation. Be sure to carefully record all of your déjà vu experiences.

One of the most emotional déjà vu episodes that I've encountered occurred while I was in Japan in the beautiful town of Kamakura. When I walked into the Engakuji Temple, which was built in 1282 and dedicated to the Rinzai sect of Zen Buddhism, the familiarity of having stood there before was overwhelming. I knew that I'd been there before. As soon as I entered the grounds, the transformation within me was palpable. Everything about me changed—the way I walked, my mannerisms, my breathing pattern, and even my eyesight... I was able to see better. It was as if a past incarnation had partially overlapped my present life.

I didn't get the feeling that I had once actually lived there; rather, I felt that I was a monk who was visiting from another temple. The aching longing that I sensed while I was there was akin to a deep homesickness, but for something I couldn't quite remember.

Exercise: Exploring Cultures, Time Periods, Historical Events, and Déjà Vu

Ask yourself the following questions and jot down the answers in your Past-life Detective Journal.

- As a child, were there particular cultures that interested you? Did you ever choose a certain one for a school project? Were there books about this subject that you enjoyed reading as a youngster?

- As an adult, have you ever studied or developed a deep curiosity about a specific culture? Did you ever spend time in a different culture that felt like home?

- If you could magically transport yourself back to a specific period in history, when would it be? Why?

- If you could be a famous person in history, whom would you pick? Why?

- Have you ever experienced déjà vu? Where were you and what was your emotional response to it?

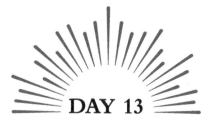

DAY 13

Dreams and Past Lives

Today we're going to discover how to gain understanding of past lives through examining our dreams. Many contain secret messages regarding not only our current lives and relationships, but also those in our far past.

It's widely accepted that dreams can offer potent insights into your life. These mysterious messages from your mind can warn you of danger, or they may contain seeds for creative inspiration. Einstein stated that his theory of relativity came to him in a dream;

in fact, he declared that many of his discoveries were the results of his nighttime reveries.

D. Scott Rogo, who was a faculty member of John F. Kennedy University in California, conducted some interesting research regarding visions of reincarnation in dreams. He placed advertisements in metaphysical-oriented magazines to elicit responses from anyone who had experienced past-life memories other than through regression methods. In his book *The Search for Yesterday*, Rogo reported that the largest group of credible recollections of past lives came from dreams.

When we're dreaming, our mind is much less likely to be confined by the limits of logic, which is why it's often the easiest way to connect with our past lives. Even people who don't believe in reincarnation have reported dreams in which they've participated in activities that took place during another time in history. This can, of course, be attributed to a recently viewed movie or a book we've just read.

However, there are some qualities that distinguish past-life dreams from ordinary ones.

Dreams that feature previous incarnations seem much more real than conventional dreams; the colors are brighter, edges and corners appear sharper, and everything seems much more vivid and clear. Frederick Lenz, a psychologist with the New School for Social Research, reports in his book *Lifetimes* that many of his subjects were aware and strongly affected when their dreams were of former lives. When past-life dreams recur, as they often do, there's usually an unresolved issue that's desperately trying to filter through to the consciousness. These dreams can be interpreted as an invitation for us to resolve that past-life conflict or difficulty.

In the next few years, I believe there will be a huge increase in the number of visions from previous incarnations that appear in our dreams, and they'll act as a filtering ground for ancient issues that are influencing our present and struggling to reach resolution.

Here's a metaphor I use to explain why our dreams are so important for resolving past-life issues. Imagine the midnight darkness of a desert. Shimmering stars punctuate the sky, as cars below wind their way along a solitary road. Most of the people driving are enjoying the silent beauty of the night; however, a few have their radios turned on, but because they're miles away from the local stations they can't pick up anything. Then from the farthest reaches of the universe, a Cosmic Radio Station (CRS) begins to broadcast to Earth.

Those with their radios on hear muffled static, as waves of increasingly higher frequencies are projected to our planet. As the intensity rises, the static also becomes louder until the signals are fine-tuned and clear. Then all mental and physical tensions ease completely, and all those who are listening hear the most exquisite music—sounds so soothing and beautiful that cares and concerns begin to fade away.

The irritations and difficulties of life dissolve, and there's a feeling of infinite peace. The very special music from the CRS stirs up a remembrance in the depths of the soul of a distant place... a place filled with an abundance of light, compassion, and fulfillment.

Right now, new frequencies and energies are flooding our planet. For many, their dreams are becoming like a turned-on radio. Because of the nonsequential, intuitive nature of dreams, you'll first "hear" many of the "CRS" frequencies through the symbols and images you perceive while sleeping. Your nighttime reveries are an untapped source of enormous potential for the planetary release that's occurring.

In the months and years ahead, many past-life visions may appear in your dreams. These new harmonics will stimulate old blockages that have resided deep within you for lifetimes. You may even feel as if your life is filled with static, and as strange as it sounds, this is a good thing because it means that your "radio" is on. (There are many people who blithely go about their seemingly static-free lives; unfortunately, because they don't have their "radios" on, they may never hear the exquisite music or experience the profound energy that you eventually will.) As these blockages are released, you'll begin to remember who you are... and the static will begin to ease, metamorphosing into a beauty you've never known before.

Your dreams can be a secret doorway into your past. Take the time to write down and record them—even if you can only recall a few snippets— because that information might help you connect to your previous lives. I recommend that you keep a notebook and pen by your bed just for this purpose. When you've amassed many fragments, try to expand them into a full scenario. This method can work well to begin to gain insights as to who you were.

Exercise:
Decoding Your Dreams

Ask yourself the following questions and jot down the answers in your Past-life Detective Journal.

- As a child, did you have any recurring dreams or nightmares?

- Have you ever had a dream that was so real you felt that you were there? What were your surroundings? Were you located in another historical period?

- Does there seem to be a theme in your dreams? For example, are you always the victim, or are you usually the antagonist or perpetrator? Are you constantly running away from something?

- Do you regularly assume a specific role in your dreams? For example, are you usually the mother, teacher, or laborer?

- Are there any people, real or imaginary, who regularly appear in your dreams? Do they usually have the same roles? How does their presence make you feel?

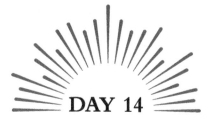

DAY 14

Remembering and Analyzing Your Dreams

Today, we continue to investigate dreams and how they can help us to understand our past-life connections.

Science has proven that everyone dreams. Even people who swear that they don't dream, in fact, do so—it's just that they don't remember their dreams, as the majority stay in our consciousness for only ten minutes. For this reason, it's valuable to quickly record your dreams before they fade from memory.

Researchers have shown that dreams occur when people are in a very light sleep state toward the end of a sleep cycle (a cycle lasts 90 minutes). Therefore, you won't feel tired later by taking some time to write down your dreams because you'll be waking up at the normal conclusion of a sleep cycle. Using a small flashlight kept beside your bed, rather than turning on the bedroom light, will enable you to fall sleep more easily after noting the content of your dreams.

Remembering your dreams is like any other skill. As you practice, you'll increase your ability to remember. You might want to note the date and time of your dreams to see if a pattern begins to emerge.

Exercise: Programming Your Dreams to Revisit Past Lives

This is an exercise that you can do just before sleep to help you remember your dreams.

As you lie down to go to sleep, take a moment to relax completely. You might begin by slowing your breath. Take long, deep breaths. Inhale fully and exhale completely.

As you begin to relax, tell yourself, "All thoughts and cares are drifting away." Imagine that you're standing beside a slow-moving river. Visualize picking up your cares one by one and placing them in the river in the kind of leaf-and-stick boats that children make. Watch each one gently float away, taking with it each and every concern. This clears your mind of interference, and you can relax even more.

Next, starting with your toes, go through your body, allowing each part to let go. For example, focus upon your right foot; breathe deeply, holding the breath for a second; and then exhale, allowing your right foot to become totally limp and free of tension. Continue until your entire body is utterly at ease. Some people report feeling so heavy that they couldn't move if they wanted to; others say that it feels like floating on a cloud.

Once you're completely relaxed, make sure that your spine is straight. Then imagine a blue light at the back of your throat, and say aloud to yourself (as the spoken word often has greater impact on the subconscious mind): "Tonight I travel to one of my past lives... and I remember my dreams." Hold this in mind with as much intensity as you can as you drift off to sleep.

Analyzing Your Dreams

See if there's any similarity between your past-life dreams and your current life. Is there someone from a previous lifetime who strikes you as very similar to someone you know now? Notice your emotions in that past life and any decisions or judgments you made. Are any patterns, habits, or fears in that life present now? For example, let's say you dream of being lost in a snowstorm and are frightened, and in your current life you always avoid being outside during harsh weather. This dream could be evidence of your past-life trauma. But remember, one clue isn't enough. You must become a past-life detective and put all the clues together to form a clear picture.

I recently had a dream that I was in a building with small rooms. Many people were crowded inside, and there was a pervading feeling of fear. The major themes were small rooms, crowding, and not feeling safe. I listed these important aspects of the dream, and the next step was to look for some correlation to my present life.

At that time we were remodeling our home, and the contents of a number of rooms were packed into just a few. It felt very crowded. In addition, due to the construction work, some of the doors were off their hinges—perhaps subconsciously I felt that our home wasn't safe. This seemed like a reasonable explanation for my dream. Then I saw the film *Schindler's List*, and I was astonished to see that the crowded rooms I'd dreamed of only nights before looked almost exactly like the rooms in the Warsaw ghetto where many Jews were crowded into before they were rounded up and sent to concentration camps. My dream had a correlation with my present life, but at the same time it provided another clue for me as I explored a past life during which I was interned in Auschwitz.

For some people, past lives appear visually and specifically in their dreams, while others wake up with no visual images but have a profound feeling or sensation.

If you've programmed your dreams as I described above and you awaken with no specific mental pictures, take a moment to notice what you're feeling. If you feel sad, expand the sadness into a story. It might go like this: "This sadness feels like the kind that a person would experience if they lost someone very close to them—perhaps a child. It doesn't feel like my child but someone else's. The little one was carefree and happy, and I wish I could have warned her not to get too close to the waterfall." When you make up your story, don't be overly concerned if it's right. The more you struggle to be correct, the more difficult it is for the images to flow from your subconscious.

Write down your stories as well as the memories of your dreams. Sometimes the stories will seem to have a life of their own and take shape without any effort. It's very important, however, to do this exercise just as you're waking up. This is the most powerful time for your subconscious to give you information about your past. Often people tell me that when they review their notebook entries and dream memories, they've been able to watch as the pieces of their reincarnation puzzle begin to fall into place.

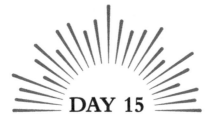

DAY 15

Using the Power of Creative Visualization

Today we are moving on to learn about past-life regression using the power of creative visualization. Embarking on a past-life odyssey not only allows you to see who you've been, but in a deeper sense, it will connect you to the true essence of your soul. The more you practice—and the more past-life experiences you become aware of and resolve—the greater balance you'll achieve in your current life.

The most important aspect is to enjoy yourself...
and you can increase your enjoyment by not being
overly serious as you examine who you were. It helps
to look at each life as a role that you performed in a
play—you're no longer that character, no more than
you're a coat that you take off when you enter your
home. You are an infinite, eternal being and every
past life is just a part you played in order to learn
and grow spiritually... in truth, the role is not who
you truly are.

Almost everyone who goes through a past-life
regression is touched by the images, memories, and
emotions that surface; and no matter how fleeting
they may be, transformative changes occur almost
mystically in the lives of those individuals. Simply
beginning to examine your past lives—even if at
first they're just snippets of memories—initiates
powerful healing and releases limitations.

As your memories from the past begin to be
revealed, you may only gain small fragments or
ephemeral images. It may feel like a subtle echo of a

recollection at the edge of your mind, but you just can't quite remember it; or you may see a quick flash of a memory, but you can't fully grasp it. Sometimes instead of a visual impression, you may have an emotional response or a visceral experience, for your body subconsciously holds the memories of all your previous lives. Be conscious of every thought, feeling, and image—no matter how seemingly insignificant—because each may offer a valuable key to unlock your past.

Also be aware that in your early attempts to discover prior incarnations, the images might be jumbled— just like trying to remember instances from your childhood.

Sometimes there's an overlap in which images from one life merge with another. For example, you might witness a Roman chariot flying through the dust and yet there's a hot-air balloon overhead. This doesn't mean that what you're seeing isn't valid; it's just an indication that two lives have collided. However, the more you practice, the clearer and less disordered the memories will become. Also, as you accumulate past-life clues and complete the following exercises, a more accurate picture will begin to unfold.

The most common method of past-life regression involves using your powers of visualization and practicing what shamans call journeying. Visualization is an excellent technique because it allows you to reach the subconscious. It's medically and scientifically recognized that visualized scenarios actually bring about psychological and even physiological changes—in some cases to almost the same degree as direct experience.

The significance of this phenomenon can be applied to past-life therapy. If you visualize a journey to a past life and resolve it, your subconscious will recognize that inner journey as a real one—and it will recognize and accept the resolution that you've come to as a real one.

When doing past-life processes, you'll become aware only of the incarnations that reflect something that you're also dealing with in your present life. Whatever lifetime you see will contain the people, situations, or issues that symbolize those in your life now. Wherever you are at any point in your current existence mirrors one or only a couple of particular past lives, and you'll usually be surrounded or closely involved with individuals from those lifetimes. In the future, you may be influenced by completely different previous incarnations.

For example, Sarah became absorbed by her spiritual path and started to become involved with her local church. She began to assist at the Sunday-morning children's group and developed a number of new friendships within the congregation. At the same time, she developed a fascination with candles and incense. In a past-life regression, she discovered that she'd been a nun in the south of France—where they'd burned many candles and used incense—and realized that her new church friends had all been nuns at the same abbey. In their shared past life, they'd cared for orphaned children. They were drawn together once again in similar circumstances in order to resolve any karmic blockages they may have accrued in their past lives. When Sarah balanced the karma from that experience, she moved on to other interests.

Contrary to skeptics of regression, rarely is anyone famous. In fact, out of the thousands of people I've regressed in my private sessions and group regressions, almost no one was a well-known figure from history. The majority are ordinary individuals facing the challenges that have emerged throughout the course of humanity: hunger, wars, migration, disease, political upheaval, and survival amid the elements. The lives that you encounter will be filled with the same obstacles that people have confronted throughout time. (And I have yet to meet the reincarnation of Cleopatra.)

To ensure that your regression is a positive experience, pick an emotionally and physically comfortable place in your home where you can do it. Select a time when you're not overwhelmed by external stresses. You may also want someone you care about and trust to be present and ready to talk to you after the process, if you feel you might need such assistance. This can be helpful not only for dealing with past-life issues that are negative, but also for sorting out the positive ones. A good discussion with a close friend can be extremely valuable for gaining a clear perspective and piecing together an entire picture from fragments of information.

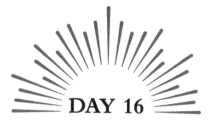

DAY 16

The Inner Voyage: A Past-life Visualization Technique

Today we are going to look at one of my favorite past-life visualization techniques—the Inner Voyage. To use this visualization technique for past-life regression, you may want to create a recording for yourself to listen to as you practice. You could also ask a friend to read aloud a script that you've created, or simply imagine yourself on this sacred journey. If you like, you can substitute "I" for "you" in the visualization. Here's a summary of the steps in The Inner Voyage.

Step 1—The Sanctuary: Relax and then imagine yourself in a peaceful place in nature. This step is essential for your ultimate outcome.

Step 2—The Transition from Present to Past: Shift out of the imagined place in nature into a neutral middle ground before actually experiencing a past life. The transition stage provides the means to enter into your distant past.

Step 3—The Past Life: This is the stage where you actually experience who you were in one of your incarnations.

Step 4—Resolving Issues: During this stage, you release your attachment to that life, enter the sanctity of the spirit world, and examine and resolve issues from that past incarnation.

Step 1: The Sanctuary

To begin your visual journey to your past, first allow yourself to become very relaxed. Then imagine going to a place in nature; this can be either a made-up setting or somewhere you've actually been where you've felt at peace. This is your sanctuary—a place where you feel safe and grounded.

If you have difficulty visualizing, as some people do, I suggest that you get a sense of being in the natural world, using your other sense organs. To do so, you might imagine the sounds around you: birds singing, a faraway waterfall, the babble of a brook, and so on. Try to really perceive what scents and physical sensations you might experience. For example, if you imagine yourself in the woods, does the aroma of fresh air and pine trees clear your head? Can you feel the warmth of the sun penetrate your body as you walk along, or perhaps as you lie stretched out on a smooth sun-baked rock?

Visualizing yourself in nature will help you become calm and serene before going on to your past-life regression. You'll feel the connection with the earth, and this provides great comfort to many people. (The sanctuary increases your feeling of safety and well-being before stepping into the past.)

Step 2: The Transition from Present to Past

Once you've imagined a place in nature, it's important to have a transition time before delving into a previous life. You'll be traveling a long way into your past, so you can think of the transition as a kind of gentle vehicle that will carry you wherever you want to go, ensuring a safe arrival with minimal culture shock. You need such a mechanism in order to let your mind and body adjust to the suspension of linear time and space. Here are some methods that can help you make a successful transition, which is the first stage to the regression exercises. Choose the technique that feels best to you.

Time Tunnel

Leave your safe place (or nature sanctuary) and walk into a time tunnel. You might count the steps or imagine getting closer and closer until you finally step into a past life.

Bridge of Time

While you're in nature, a bridge appears before you. Climb up its ascending steps high above the clouds. As you continue your journey, descend down the bridge back through the clouds and into a past life.

River of Time

Climb into a small boat lined with soft pillows. Lie down and watch the clouds overhead as the boat travels of its own volition through the river of time, taking you to a past life.

Cosmic Elevator

Step into the cosmic elevator. Every floor number on the lighted panel represents a different lifetime. You can either push a button or wait for the elevator to stop. When the doors open, you enter a past life.

Mystical Door

Imagine what the mystical door looks like, feels like, and even what sound it makes when you knock on it. When it opens, a past life is revealed.

Time Machine

A time machine appears in your sanctuary. You enter it and the machine lifts up into the clouds. When it descends, you're in a past life. You can even have a panel inside that shows you the exact date you've arrived in.

Magical Theater

Imagine that you've entered a large and beautiful theater where a number of movies are showing.

Each of these films allows you to explore a past life. You can choose to enter by stepping into the screen, or you may decide to sit back and watch your past life from the safe perspective of a comfortable theater seat. Additionally, you can watch actors portray your past lives just as if you were in an actual theater.

The Doorkeeper

In your safe place in nature, you encounter a wise and gentle being. This is the Doorkeeper, a past-life guide who knows all about you, loves you very much, and is able to safely guide you wherever you need to go. You can ask this being any questions about your past; and this wise being can lead you back to a previous life, into a future one, or even to another realm. Your kind guide might also present you with a gift that will be useful in your past-life journeys.

There are endless variations on these exercises. Try them out to see which ones work best for you. Here are a few more ideas:

- Magical Time Bubble

- Transporter (think *Star Trek*)

- Mystical Train

- Through the Vortex (recall *Sliders* or *Stargate*)

- Quantum Leap

- Small Plane that Travels Through Time

- Closets of Abilities or Room of Costumes

- Bazaar with Tents that Open to Different Realms (similar to *Harry Potter*)

- Book of Life (with moving pictures)

- Ancient Library of Time

Step 3: The Past Life

After you successfully transition from your sanctuary in nature, the next step is to actually visualize a previous life. Once you've gone through a metamorphosis into your past-life body, take a moment to look down at your feet and notice where you're standing. Observe the shoes you're wearing or the coverings on your feet. Do they appear to be male or female, young or old? Ask yourself, *Am I indoors or outdoors?* If you're outside, what does the landscape look like? Be aware of noises, smells, and physical sensations; most of all, be cognizant of your emotional state. Once you begin to get a sense of where you are—and who you are—you can explore that life. (At any time you desire, you can immediately slip out of this past life, and return to the present time.)

Step 4: Resolving Issues

Once you've completed your exploration, imagine yourself floating out of that body and entering a beautiful, peaceful spirit world where you can review the past incarnation you've just experienced. While in the safety of the ethereal realm, you're also able to release old patterns, forgive others or accept self-forgiveness, and reconnect with the Creator.

To do this, first review the past life you've just visited with an air of sacred detachment. Understand that everything you've experienced in that incarnation was for your development as a soul. Ask yourself, *What did I learn during the turning points in that life, and what was the meaning of each event?* When you feel complete, imagine that you're radiating love and joy to that lifetime from your vantage point in the realm of spirit.

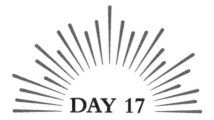

DAY 17

The Inner Voyage Meditation

Today we are going to do the Inner Voyage Meditation, which is an example of how to put together all four of the Inner Voyage steps that we learned about yesterday.

The Inner Voyage Meditation

Start by getting your body into a relaxed position, either sitting or reclining. Now take some very deep breaths. With each breath you take and each sound you hear, you become more and more relaxed.

Put your attention on your left foot and feel it completely let go. Allow a delicious wave of relaxation to slowly roll from your feet up through your hips to your torso, stretching through your arms and hands, and up and out of the top of your head. Your entire body is now relaxed, warm, and comfortable. Take one deep breath, totally surrender, and let go.

Imagine that you're walking across a field. It's a sunny day and you're filled with the deep scent of lush summer grasses. You hear the soft drone of insects and the merry songs of birds... these sounds fill the air with a soothing, rhythmic cadence. A mist begins to rise from the field and stillness fills the air. In the distance, you hear a gentle river lapping against the bank. As you approach, the mist becomes very thick. At the water's edge, you notice a sturdy bridge crossing it. This is the Bridge of Time.

The mist has become so thick that you can't make out the other side of the bridge; in fact, you can only see a few feet in front of you as you step onto it. With each step you take, you know you're nearing one of your past lives.

Count slowly from 1 to 10. When you reach the end, you'll step off the bridge at a time long ago, before you came into your present body. Although you can't see, you begin to feel yourself changing as you shapeshift into the body that you occupied in a previous incarnation. Begin now: 1-2-3-4... with each step you take, the swirling, mystical mist seems to embrace you with warmth and love... 5-6-7... you're aware of a loving presence guiding and protecting your every step... 8-9... the fog is beginning to thin, the end of the bridge is near... 10... step off the bridge.

You've arrived in one of your past lives. The mist has completely cleared. Look down at your feet. Are they the feet of a man or a woman? Are they young- or old-looking? Are you outside or inside? What surface are you standing on? Sand? Stone? Tile? Wooden floor? Grass? What covering do you have on your feet? What type of clothing are you wearing? Do you feel more male or female? Are you young, old, or middle-aged? Look around and note your surroundings. Are you in the country or the city? If there are any buildings, pay attention to the architecture. Are there any people nearby? If there are, listen to them speaking. What language does it sound like? Is there anyone who resembles a person from your present life? As you wander around and perceive this life, tune in to your emotions. How does this life feel? You have a few minutes to explore. Be willing to use your imagination. You may begin now.

Go to a time in this life that was very significant or important to you. You have a short while to experience what's happening and to determine how you feel about these circumstances. Continue to move forward in time in the past life that you're exploring... go onward to the moment when you're about to shed your body and pass over to the spirit world. How did you die? Was it slowly or suddenly? What people were around you? Were you reluctant or glad to go? From a spiritual view, the process of dying is seldom recognized as a painful event, and there's usually a great sigh of relief once you realize that you've passed over. It's like returning home after a long absence. You have a minute to observe this event in your past life. You may do this now.

Go forward into the spirit world. From your perspective in the spirit world, what did you learn from the past life? Were there any fears or concerns from there that are still present in your life today?

As you discover where these fears originated, you now know that they aren't real, and it's simple to release them. Just let go. You know that you can create your life in the present to be exactly the way you want it. You can choose freely without programming from other lives.

Now it's time to let all of this fade away and return to your current life. Just let the past life fade away... just drift away.

As you move closer to normal waking awareness, you feel strong and empowered. You've stepped into your far past with courage and have looked at who and what you were. With this examination, your present life is enhanced and you've taken a step closer to the divinity within you. In the future, you're free to explore any past life, and the knowledge you gain creates the space for your life to be more fulfilling and whole.

Count from 1 to 5. When you reach 5, you'll be totally awake and aware... 1-2... your body is healthy and strong... 3... more and more alert... 4... your eyes feel as if they've been bathed in fresh, cooling spring water... 5... wide awake and feeling great. Open your eyes now. Stretch and enjoy the beauty of the day.

You can use The Inner Voyage Meditation again and again. You might want to try it right before bed, as this will encourage past-life recall in your dreams.

DAY 18

How to Heal Past-life Blockages with Regression: Method 1

One of the main benefits of regression therapy is that it can finally free you of the hindrances that have been holding you back throughout many lifetimes. However, for this to occur you need to learn how to resolve those blockages. Today and in the next two chapters we'll discover a number of simple exercises we can do alone or with a friend to finally unravel the lingering issues that have been obstructing our lives. (I suggest that you try several or all of the exercises to find out which ones work best for you.)

Method 1

People have often asked me, "What if I do the processes and come up with a lifetime that's scary… or what if I have a past-life nightmare?" Instead of shutting down or suppressing these emotions, choose to feel them—when you do so, the fear will dissipate. For example, when you see an action thriller at the movie theater, you pay to be frightened; you're going out of your way to create an intense experience for yourself. There are times in life when we choose to be scared, but we're not overwhelmed because it was by choice.

Don't be afraid of the emotions you might encounter when you get in touch with a past life. Choose them. No one would attend an orchestral performance if only one note was to be played. A symphony needs thousands of tones—high points and low. Life is like that, too. Enjoy all your emotions and think of each one as a precious note in your unique musical composition. As you experience a past life, relish and explore each feeling that arises.

If you find yourself stuck in an emotion during a past-life journey, don't deny it or try to get rid of it; instead, move toward it and choose it. See yourself confronting that feeling and letting it flow all around you. Exaggerate it. For instance, if you discover a lifetime in which you were devastated by the death of your lover, instead of trying to deny or repress the grief—which is what you did at the time—let yourself feel even sadder.

Go to the center of that sorrow. Find the spot in your body where it resides, and allow yourself to enter into it. This will enable you to begin releasing the issues that have been creating barriers for you.

When I began conducting past-life therapy seminars, many people would cry or sob during the processes—sometimes very dramatically. I assumed this was an important step toward the ultimately positive results they would achieve. Then when I led a seminar in Vancouver, Canada, and nobody cried uncontrollably, I was distraught, thinking my techniques hadn't worked. However, I was astonished to receive numerous letters afterward from participants of that seminar claiming positive results. I figured it was a fluke, but the same thing occurred in my next seminar and has continued ever since.

In my past-life seminars today, almost no one becomes emotional even though very dramatic, positive results are always reported. As I began to investigate this phenomenon, I realized that instead of externalizing and amplifying their emotions, people were going to the source of their feelings… and truly embracing them. As strange as it sounds, sometimes dramatizing your emotions can actually keep you separate from them.

By finding the place in your body where the emotion exists and going into it, you can release it at its roots. This is an exercise you can do if you begin to feel any uncomfortable emotions during your past-life regressions.

As I just mentioned, if you encounter a previous incarnation in which you discover a very difficult event or face some challenging emotions, begin by traveling throughout your body to locate the feeling associated with the traumatic event. (There's always a sensation in your body that's associated with an emotion.) For example, your chest might feel constricted during sadness and your shoulders might tighten during anger. However, not everyone experiences emotions in the same way.

Once you've located the emotion you're feeling, focus your entire attention on that part of your body and intensify the sensation. If you feel a constriction in your chest, make it tighter. Feel it more. As you do so, identify what shape the emotion/sensation seems to be.

The tightness in the chest associated with sadness might seem pear-shaped, with the smaller end of the pear pointing downward. As you focus on the area, also observe how large the sensation is. The pear might seem about six inches wide and eight inches long. Then notice if it has a color. (It's not mere coincidence that people associate particular colors with certain emotions: "She's in the pink," "He's feeling blue," "I'm having a black day," "He saw red," and so on.)

Continue to ask yourself these questions:

- If there was a place in my body associated with this emotion, where might it be? (Sometimes the sensation will shift to various spots in the body. Follow it wherever it goes.)

- If the sensation had a shape, what would it look like?

- If the sensation had a size, how big would it be?

- If the sensation had a color, what color would it be?

Keep on intensifying what you're feeling. Often the color, shape, size, and location change as you're doing this exercise, but continue moving into your emotions, rather than away from them. Just practicing these steps is usually enough to begin releasing the uncomfortable feelings that arose during your past-life experiences. What you resist persists… and when you quit resisting what you're feeling, it can dissolve.

Sometimes when you do this exercise, memories from another past life will emerge spontaneously. In the same way that a temper tantrum thrown at age 20 may be the result of a temper tantrum thrown under similar circumstances at age 3, so the past-life trauma that you're working with may have its source in yet another, similar lifetime. So don't be surprised if you find yourself catapulted from one former incarnation to another. It's beneficial because with each time-jump you're getting even closer to the source of your present-life difficulty. Doing this exercise can allow the undesirable emotions and the past-life blockage to disappear.

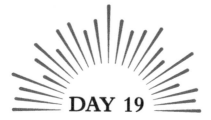

DAY 19

How to Heal Past-life Blockages with Regression: Methods 2 and 3

Today we are going to find out how to let go of a particular view of a past-life by detaching from it or by seeing it from a completely different perspective.

Method 2

If you find yourself in a past-life memory that holds very uncomfortable emotions, a good way to deal with it is to imagine that you're floating above the scene and just observe it.

When you detach from a situation, you can observe it from a greater, more objective perspective. Beryl experienced a lifetime in which her husband died of an infection he contracted while working in their garden. In her regression, she felt tremendous sadness tinged with guilt over her loss. The sadness was for the loss of her husband; the guilt was due to the fact that she'd been capable of completing the garden work but told her husband that she wasn't strong enough to do it. Although of course it wasn't her fault, she felt culpable, and that emotion had permeated her present life.

When she detached from the scene and floated above it to gain an expanded perspective, she saw that her intense love for her husband was sometimes to the detriment of her children. She often put aside their needs in order to spend more time with her spouse. After his death, she began to nurture her kids more and give them the attention and love they needed. When she removed herself from the picture, she was able to come to terms with her husband's death and understand that everything has a purpose, even if she didn't realize it at the time.

When you detach from a scene, you can float above it or watch it as if you were viewing a movie. If it's very traumatic, you can observe yourself looking at the scene as a way of further detaching from the situation.

Another technique I often suggest is to fast-forward the incident at high speed, like an old Charlie Chaplin film. Then run it backward at high speed. For example, if you find yourself running and falling off a cliff, see yourself running and falling very fast and then flipping up off the ground, soaring back to the top of the cliff, and running backward! This exercise, which can make any seemingly distressful event humorous, can help you detach from it.

Yet another way to remove yourself from an uncomfortable past life is to make it seem silly. A client who had always felt intimidated by men came to me for help. She was a mature, responsible woman but as soon as she was near a man, she began to act in a meek, childlike way. Having regressed to a life in which she had a strict, disciplinarian father, she saw that whenever she was with men, she activated the memory of being a timid little girl from that past life. During her regression, she arrived at a point where her father was giving her a stern dressing-down. I told her to imagine him standing in front of her wearing red spotted pants and a silly hat as people walked by and laughed. Suddenly she, too, was laughing, and she was no longer a submissive young girl. This session completely changed her attitude toward men.

Detaching from a past-life scene helps you understand that every lifetime you have allows you to grow—and that everything you encounter is important for your evolution as a soul. When you observe a past life with an objective point of view, you see that Spirit is interested not so much in your comfort as in your personal growth, even if it means going through difficult, painful experiences.

Method 3

A technique for resolving past-life situations that involve another person is to imagine that you're jumping into the awareness or the body of that individual. See the entire situation from his or her point of view. When you do so, you almost always forgive the other's actions because you recognize that you would have reacted in the same way.

An interesting example is the case of Charlotte. She'd been quarreling with her younger sister seemingly since her sister was born. The fighting had continued into adulthood, and their arguments were having a negative effect on the entire family, as they tried to get other family members to agree with their points of view. Charlotte became aware that these altercations were becoming increasingly counterproductive and affecting many areas of her life.

She attended a past-life workshop I gave in New Zealand and recalled a life in which she was an accounting clerk in Denmark, and her present-life sister was her demanding and argumentative employer. In the regression, she took my suggestion of seeing the world through her employer's eyes. Instantly, she understood that her employer had very severe back pain that made his every move painful. Because of his debilitating pain, he was continually in a foul mood and treated his employees badly.

With this new understanding, Charlotte began to feel compassion for her employer/sister. (It's interesting to note that her sister in her present life also had a back injury.) Charlotte reported that she saw her sister a few days after the seminar and was astonished to find that there was much less animosity between them. Their relationship has continued to grow closer.

Resolving past-life blockages is one of the most rewarding kinds of work you can do. Many of my clients have reported a greater sense of exhilaration and joy than they'd ever experienced before… but it can be a rough and rocky road while you're in the process. Share your challenges with someone who cares about you, or seek professional assistance if you think you need it, and know that what awaits you is more than worth it.

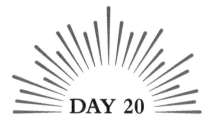

DAY 20

How to Heal Past-life Blockages with Regression: Method 4

The most powerful technique to resolve an uncomfortable past-life issue is to change the circumstances of that life until it feels comfortable or enjoyable, and this is our topic for today. I believe that you can actually change the past. If this is too far-fetched for you to accept, then imagine that you're altering the images stored in your brain. As you transform them, you also change the associated limiting beliefs.

I believe that the future and the past are malleable, and from the viewpoint of physics, this isn't a totally far-fetched idea. According to scientists, time is a function of gravity and it can shorten or lengthen depending on how far away you are from the gravitational pull of the Earth. I don't know whether this scientific fact applies to the metaphysical notion that time is an illusion, but it does give credence to the idea that time isn't as we usually perceive it.

Personally, I've experienced profound changes in my own life—and in the lives of others—simply by going into past lives and altering the events. Whether you believe, as I do, that you're actually altering your past or if you're just imagining that the past is different isn't important. What is important is that as a result of these changes, your life transforms in positive and powerful ways.

There are many cases of individuals regressing to a past life and healing the wounds that occurred at the time (and continue to play out in their present life) simply by changing the memories they'd associated with that event (or by changing the meaning they gave to it). That past-life healing then transforms their present-day lives. In other words, when you heal your past—by changing those past events—you can create a balanced and harmonious future.

Changing the memories of a previous incarnation and, as a consequence, creating a better outcome for yourself is the most compelling method for resolution that I know of. When you recreate your past, you no longer need to view yourself as a victim—you can take control of your life. And you always have the power to create an empowering past! Accept the soul growth that each life offers and at the same time, create a past that supports you and gives you joy. On a soul level, each lifetime was perfect for your evolution, but at the same time, former experiences don't need to repeat in your future. It's never too late to have a blissful past. However, if it seems too philosophical to think about really changing old events, just consider it as altering the past that dwells within your mind. All the memories—and all the associated limiting beliefs and negative programming—exist in your mind. Change your mind and change your life.

Here's a personal example from my life that shows the step-by-step mechanics of how to recast past-life memories.

When my daughter, Meadow, was younger, I asked her if I could try a new relaxation technique on her before I practiced it on my clients. I needed to hold her wrist, but as I did so, she said, "Mom, you know I don't like to have my wrists touched. In fact, I can't even look at my wrists because when I see the veins I get squeamish."

I hadn't been aware of this before but proceeded with the relaxation process. Once she was relaxed, I thought I'd take the opportunity to see if I could get to the source of her difficulty.

I said, "Imagine a situation that might relate to your wrists." (Children, incidentally, can usually regress very easily into past lives, but adults often develop a buffer to their intuition, making it more difficult to be regressed. However, I don't suggest regressing any children until they are of consenting age.)

"Mom, I see a desert. I live in the desert." "Are you male or female?" "I'm a young man. I have a religious belief that I feel strongly about. It's a good belief, and I want to tell everyone about it because I know it will help them. I'm now in a small village preparing to talk to people about this new belief. They don't want to know about it—in fact, they're getting very angry. Oh no!"

"What is it?"

"They're tying me up. They've cut my wrists… I'm watching the blood slowly flow out of my body. I'm tied up so I can't stop it. I'm dying!"

"You can change this experience," I told her calmly. "You can replay it but give it a positive outcome."

"Okay. I'm replaying it… I've traveled across the desert to tell the villagers about my new religion.

Everyone who greets me is happy to meet me and seems really interested in talking and finding out about my beliefs. When I leave the village, I've made many good friends."

"How do you feel?"

"I feel great. It feels good to know that I can really tell people how I feel."

All this occurred in about 20 minutes. My daughter came back from her experience feeling refreshed and rejuvenated. I asked her to look at the veins on her wrists, and she was amazed that she could now look at them without feeling queasy.

Up until that point, she'd always been hesitant to say how she truly felt about anything. In fact, she was probably the least opinionated person I had ever known. But now a remarkable thing occurred. Meadow began to tell people how she felt about things and to share her personal points of view. This was something that she'd never done before! The

Gulf War broke out soon afterward, and Meadow called all the students in her class and asked them to march against the war with her. To me, this was a minor miracle. I believe that our one 20-minute session made all the difference.

Some people are concerned that if they change the past, they'll negatively affect the present. They'll ask, "What if I change the past and then my mother never meets my father. Will I still exist?" Such questions are interesting to me, philosophically, but in my experience, changing a traumatic past life always has a positive effect on everyone. When you clear an emotional blockage from your energy field, you create a resonance that deeply impacts you and others for the best. You can change the past. Just shifting the images in your brain associated with limiting beliefs has a beneficial and empowering effect on life.

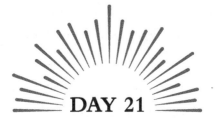

DAY 21

Looking Forward: Time and Future Lives

Today we are going to explore the concept of time and our how our perceptions of this phenomenon affect our lives.

As a small child, I sat forlornly on a rusty swing one foggy morning. My parents were having violent, physical arguments, and I was having a hard time coping with it all. Suddenly I turned my head around, quickly looking behind myself. I thought I'd sensed someone approaching, but no one was there. Then I remember a deep calmness and a sense of belonging settling over me. I no longer felt alone. After that point, although I didn't like my parents' fights, I no longer felt devastated after each one as I had before. Something had changed.

This memory had been completely forgotten until some 30 years later, when I was endeavoring to go back in time during a meditation in order to visit myself as a small child. In my visualization, I popped out of a time tunnel to 1955 to find myself comforting a very young Denise as she sat slumped on a rusty swing. I told her that I loved her unconditionally. I let her know that she had some tough times ahead, but she would make it and her future would be wonderful. As I spoke to her, she straightened up and it seemed that a heavy weight had been lifted from her spirit.

Coming back into the present time, I was astonished. Not only had I traveled back and visited my younger self—which of course anyone can practice doing—but the amazing thing was that as a small child in 1955, I remembered the visit! I don't recall someone talking to me that foggy morning, but I do remember sensing that someone who cared for me was by my side. And even though I couldn't see who it was, I knew that I didn't need to feel lonely anymore. It was a remarkable experience—I know that I indeed visited myself, and it had made an enormous difference in my life.

I also believe that not only can you visit your younger self to provide solace and love, but you can also call upon your spirit beyond the present to bring advice and guidance—based on what you've learned—in the future.

One of the many objections to this theory is the idea that time is fixed and can't be altered. However, time isn't an absolute. It's an infinite eternity, arbitrarily divided into portions called centuries, years, months, weeks, days, hours, seconds, and so on. In the past, we thought of time as steady and unchanging. I believe that the more you explore the universes within yourself—through meditation or other spiritual practices—the more fluid the passage of time becomes. You can actually perceive it speeding up or slowing down.

When you're involved in something creative, time flies and an hour seems like a blink of an eye. By contrast, when you're waiting for a friend who's an hour late, time seems to stretch for an eternity.

You can speed it up or slow it down subjectively. This is what I call entering hyper-time, an expression I coined because it most accurately describes this phenomenon. *Merriam-Webster's Collegiate Dictionary* defines the prefix "hyper" as "that is or exists in a space of more than three dimensions." Entering hyper-time is literally stepping into "time that dwells beyond the three dimensions."

Given the current laws that govern our physical world, it should be impossible to alter minutes and seconds in such a manner. But what if time really is fluid? What if it contracts and expands in a rhythmically pulsating universe? What if time is a function of our perception? Imagine that we can dramatically shift it and enter into the timeless Source from which all awareness emanates. Suppose we could travel to dimensionless regions where time and space are born? Given these suppositions, we could in fact alter time and even our own view of reality. I believe that these notions are true and that each and every one of us is both the perceiver and definer of time.

We're constantly changing not just our present, but our past and our future as well, from any given point in time. The universe is a fluctuating ocean of consciousness with all time occurring simultaneously. We're intimately connected in this sea of awareness. When you release an old blockage through changing your perception of the past, it's like a pebble dropped in a still pool whose ripples are felt at the farthest shore. Not only does it help you, but your immediate family members and friends are also affected positively by the "ripples," and so is everyone else on the planet who shares your frequencies... even if they don't know you.

Some people find it valuable to visit their upcoming lives or have their future selves come back through time and space in order to offer advice and guidance based on the knowledge they've gained. This is also an excellent way to assist your ability to manifest your dreams by projecting what you desire into the future. Because the time/space veil is thinning, it's becoming easier to travel in your meditations not only to the past but also to approaching events. Some people find that their inner confidence is renewed after they've witnessed destined triumphs that have yet to be realized. Others discover that they can avoid a difficult future by observing possibilities that haven't yet unfolded and making corrections today.

Sometimes individuals are concerned with how they'll cope if they see something truly terrible in their future or in a loved one's destiny. Tomorrow is as malleable as the past, and what you see is only a probability—and fortunately, you're in a position to make alterations.

Exercise: Future-life Meditation

The process used to travel to future lives is similar to what's used to access past lives. The following meditation will help you get started.

First allow yourself to become very relaxed, and picture a favorite place in nature. You might imagine yourself leaning against a willow tree as you listen to a bubbling stream nearby. Allow your entire body to become calm as you fill each and every part of yourself with tranquility. Know that every breath is enabling you to become even more comfortable. Imagine that your guide or angel is close at hand. You're at peace with the universe and are surrounded in infinite love.

Imagine that you're engulfed in a sphere of white light. You're safe and protected. As you're sitting in nature, day turns to night. One by one the stars come out, and the entire sky becomes filled with shimmering lights. A particular star draws your attention. As you gaze at it, it becomes brighter and brighter and slowly begins to float down from the sky, moving toward you.

As the star grows closer, you can see that it's actually an orb-shaped vehicle made of light and sound. It looks like a large, luminous bubble. You know this is a time machine.

You step inside and feel comforted by the lush, cocoon-like interior. Quietly, with only the softest hum, the vehicle lifts from the earth and begins to gently ascend. As you settle back into the inviting cushions, you observe the entire canopy of stars through the windows.

You feel the vehicle floating back to the earth. As you step out of your time machine, you find yourself by a beautiful, still pool. As you gaze into it, you begin to have visions. You see who you are in a future life. Notice whether you're a male or female and if any people look similar to your present-day friends or family members. Scan your future life and look for the area of greatest conflict. You're free to change the scene you're observing. In addition, see if there's anything in your present life that you can do to avert this future scenario. Surround the entire scene with love, and return to your time machine.

Begin to bring yourself to normal waking consciousness. You understand that all you've seen of your future was for your highest good, and you know that you're making the necessary adjustments in your present life in order to create an exciting, fulfilling future.

Afterword

I believe that there are countless dimensions coexisting with our reality, and we can be aware of them by adjusting an inner dial. Just as there are numerous radio stations flooding our homes and offices—but we can't hear them unless we have our radios on—we need only to find our inner dial, turn it on, and tune in; then we'll touch the Light.

Most people think of heaven as the place they go to when they die. We subconsciously think of it as somewhere way up above the clouds, but heaven, or our spiritual home, isn't in the sky. It's here, right now—a dimension coexisting with our physical reality. One way you can know that you're close to that dimension is through synchronicity.

For example, when you think of something and it happens, you need it and it suddenly appears, or you think of someone and he or she calls. The closer you get to that dimension, the faster your thoughts become manifest in the physical world.

There's nothing out there that isn't you. Because of the linear way that we perceive reality, I don't think we can ever understand this intellectually, communicate it verbally, or even write about it in a comprehensive way. However, I believe that deep inside, we all do know this and we've all had glimpses of this feeling. Even in the most fulfilled human being, there's a longing, a yearning, and a remembering of that exquisite place of oneness and unity.

Each and every part of the universe is a part of you, and you're the most astonishing blend imaginable. But most of us have forgotten because we usually identify only with our bodies and feel separate from all the other parts of ourselves. Sometimes we identify with our children or even our possessions (a man will run into a burning building to rescue valuables because in that moment, he's identifying himself more with his material possessions than with his body). In fact, you're living in a miraculous ocean of energy, and each part of that powerful flow is you. You might imagine all these parts as making up a gigantic orchestra of energy. When there's a harmonization of all these aspects, a vibration is created that resonates throughout the universe.

This is what my Native American ancestors meant when they talked about being in "right relation" with all things. It means to honor and respect the livingness in all things. Cherish the animal or plant that gives you life... revere all that's around you. Listen—really listen—and acknowledge the reality of your neighbors, for they aren't separate from you. They are you!

Living in right relation with all things means living in harmony with all other elements of the collective Spirit. One way to do so is to unconditionally accept the reality of others. This also means moving toward acceptance of all parts of yourself, especially the aspects that you've judged negatively and even what you embodied in your past lives. Being in right relation signifies helping others wherever you can without expecting anything in return. It implies acting with compassion toward all the life force.

Know that there's no less energy in your computer than in the beautiful apple tree growing outside your window. Honor, accept, and love the life that's all around you, for it's all you in different forms. Whatever you judge sets you further along the path of separateness; whatever you love allows the orchestra of all your parts (which in its totality is the Creator) to vibrate and sing with joy throughout the universe. As the shackles of the past loosen their hold through your exploration of your previous incarnations, may you find true peace. May joy abound in your life beyond your greatest expectations!

About the Author

Denise Linn is an internationally renowned teacher in the field of self-development. She has written 19 books, which are available in 29 languages, including the bestseller *Sacred Space* and the award-winning *Feng Shui for the Soul*. Denise has appeared in numerous documentaries and television shows worldwide and is the founder of the Red Lotus Woman's Mystery School, which offers professional certification programmes.

www.deniselinn.com